Magical Beginnings,

Enchanted Lives

THE SEVEN SPIRITUAL LAWS FOR PARENTS

HEALING THE HEART

EVERYDAY IMMORTALITY

THE LORDS OF THE LIGHT

ON THE SHORES OF ETERNITY

HOW TO KNOW GOD

THE SOUL IN LOVE

THE CHOPRA CENTER HERBAL HANDBOOK
(with David Simon)

GROW YOUNGER, LIVE LONGER
(with David Simon)

THE DEEPER WOUND

THE CHOPRA CENTER COOKBOOK
(with David Simon and Leanne Backer)

THE ANGEL IS NEAR

THE DAUGHTERS OF JOY

GOLF FOR ENLIGHTENMENT

SOULMATE

THE SPONTANEOUS FULFILLMENT OF DESIRE

THE BOOK OF SECRETS

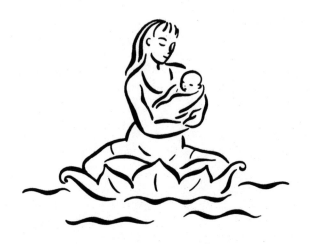

A HOLISTIC GUIDE TO

PREGNANCY AND CHILDBIRTH

Magical Beginnings, Enchanted Lives

Deepak Chopra, M.D.,

DAVID SIMON, M.D. & VICKI ABRAMS, C.C.E., I.B.C.L.C.

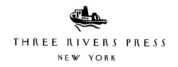

THREE RIVERS PRESS

NEW YORK

A note on gender: We have elected to alternate pronoun gender when referring to the unborn baby. We will use *he, his,* and *him* in odd-numbered chapters and *she, hers,* and *her* in the introduction and even-numbered chapters.

Library of Congress Cataloging-in-Publication Data
Chopra, Deepak.
Magical beginnings, enchanted lives : a holistic guide to
pregnancy and childbirth / Deepak Chopra, David Simon,
and Vicki Abrams.—1st ed.
Includes index.
1. Pregnancy.   2. Childbirth.   3. Medicine, Ayurvedic.
4. Meditation.   5. Yoga, Haòtha.   I. Simon, David, 1951–
II. Abrams, Vicki.   III. Title.
RG525.C475 2005
618.2'44—dc22   2004019702

ISBN 0-517-70220-7

Printed in the United States of America

Design by Lauren Dong and Jennifer Ann Daddio

10   9   8   7   6   5   4   3   2   1

First Edition

To the children of humanity,
whose innocent hands hold
the future of our world

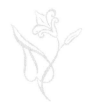

Contents

Introduction
A CONSCIOUS PREGNANCY   1

Chapter 1
CREATING A BABY   17

Chapter 2
WOMB ECOLOGY   43

Chapter 3
NOURISHMENT FOR TWO   71

Chapter 4
MAINTAINING YOUR BALANCE   95

Contents

Chapter 5
WEATHERING THE CHANGES   127

Chapter 6
PARTNERS IN LOVE   151

Chapter 7
THE BIRTHING JOURNEY   175

Chapter 8
NURTURING MOTHER AND BABY   235

Chapter 9
FATHERHOOD FUNDAMENTALS   273

Conclusion
HEALING THE WORLD ONE CHILD AT A TIME   295

Glossary of Terms   301

Suggested Reading   307

Index   309

Magical Beginnings,
Enchanted Lives

INTRODUCTION

A Conscious Pregnancy

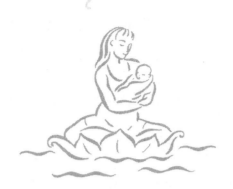

*T*he creative impulse of life is the most powerful force in the universe. Mysterious and inexplicable, it is more substantial than matter, subtler than thought, and more enduring than time. Since the beginning of humanity we have sought explanations of how life emerges from inanimate elements. Despite the unraveling of the genetic code, life remains as much a mystery now as in ancient times.

The perennial wisdom traditions tell us that archetypal gods and goddesses brought us forth in their image so that we could re-create and honor them in our image. Science ponders the organizing principles that seduce atoms into molecules, molecules into complex biochemicals, and biochemicals into self-replicating systems. Do life-forms exist to reproduce DNA molecules or do DNA molecules exist to reproduce life-forms? Whether you see the universe as personal or impersonal, from a spiritual or a scientific perspective, you have to marvel at the animating vital force that orchestrates the creation of all living beings.

The universe is re-created in every individual life. Birth and death are merely parentheses in the never-ending story of creation. Each human birth holds the promise of adventure, drama, love, and loss. In the process of creation, the universal ocean of love temporarily flows in rivers of individuality seeking their return to the source. Your baby's conception and birth are the first pages of a new tale—the first steps on her path through this world of infinite possibilities.

Our book, *Magical Beginnings, Enchanted Lives,* is a celebration of birth—an exultation of each flower of individuality that blooms on the tree of life. The magic and the mystery of life's creative process enable each individual and each new generation to recapitulate the entire history of life while seeking ever-new expressions. As your baby takes her first breath and the umbilical cord is cut, she becomes an individual. She separates from your body and formally begins her journey of self-discovery. Intuition and research clearly show us that long before your baby is launched through the birth canal, she has begun exploring her own personhood.

Your baby's sense of self-awareness dawns early as she

grows inside your watery womb. As soon as her sensory awareness develops, she perceives and responds to subtle sounds, sensations, sights, tastes, and smells from inside your body. Your interpretations of the world filter through your body to your unborn baby. She readily learns to associate her experiences with feelings and emotions and has pleasures and discomforts of her own. For nine months while your baby is linked to you as her mother ship, she is continually tapping into your database of the world. Your baby learns to associate sensory impulses with feelings and identifies those that bring nourishment and those that feel toxic. Life learning clearly begins before birth.

This book is designed for pregnant women, their partners, women who wish to become pregnant, and for anyone who wants to participate in the wondrous process of bringing new life into this world. We have also sought to include information for people whose work addresses the common childhood problems of modern life—teachers, counselors, therapists, and health providers will find this book invaluable. This is not simply a book about fetal health, for we believe that the knowledge provided can improve the health of society at large. The suffering, depression, and crime that surround us each day are strong statements about a loss of balance between body, mind, and spirit. This loss often starts at the very beginning of a life before birth. The tendency toward a balanced state of health and wholeness and the tendency to lose this intrinsic but delicate balance are both present in seed form at the moment of conception.

The book has been incubating in our hearts and minds for many years. In caring for people at the Chopra Center with a wide range of imbalances and illnesses, we have learned that experiences are metabolized into biology. We can heal our bodies by making different choices. Many of our patients and guests express the wish that they had received guidance on living a balanced life as children. Through extensive research we became aware that developing human beings learn about life and the world even while in the womb, and the choices made by their parents have lasting effects. To put this knowledge into practice, we developed the Magical Beginnings birth education program and have trained prenatal educators around the world. Our experience in teaching Magical Beginnings to pregnant couples at the Chopra Center has convinced us that the principles and practices presented in this book can profoundly enhance the experience of pregnancy and birth for both the parents and the baby.

Experiences long before birth affect and mold personality. A baby can show the signs of stress even before he or she is born. Feelings and desires are shaped by our intrauterine experiences. Science has demonstrated that every wisp of experience is metabolized into the substance of our minds and bodies, both before and after we are born into this world. Nourishing experiences from conception through life are transformed into healthy bodies and healthy minds, while toxic experiences create unhealthy ones.

Health is not the mere absence of disease; it is a state of physical, psychological, emotional, and spiritual well-being.

We can even go further and define health as a higher state of consciousness, in which we recognize that the same field of intelligence that underlies our life underlies every living being. In a true state of health, we become incapable of hurting others or ourselves. To achieve this state it is important that we feel loved, nourished, secure, contented, and happy, right from the beginning. From the moment of conception, the unborn baby experiences the thoughts and actions of her mother. This is because mind and body are inseparably one. Wherever a thought goes, a molecule follows. The impulses in our minds are instantly translated into a palette of neurochemicals. These chemicals communicate with cells and tissues throughout our body. The unborn baby is a part of her mother's body. Therefore, a mother's thoughts, emotions, and feelings translate into molecules that enter into the body of her fetus.

You and your baby are continuously sharing each other's molecules and experiences. This dynamic exchange of information and these chemical messengers are the codes of communication between your heart and mind and the heart and mind of your unborn baby. The start of a rich emotional life begins as early as conception. The choices that you make as a mother are key to providing the best beginning, and your expanded awareness is the key to making the best choices. In this book, we hope to bring into the awareness of all parents the understanding that their choices, interpretations, and experiences before, during, and after pregnancy play an essential role in the development of healthy and happy children. By making nourishing choices, you can ensure that your baby is receiving the basic elements to create a healthy body, mind, and spirit.

In this book we regularly refer to the profound insights of the ancient wisdom sciences of Ayurveda. This five-thousand-year-old system of natural medicine with its origins in ancient India reminds us that human beings are, in essence, spiritual. Acknowledging this, we can begin to grasp the sacred responsibility of conceiving, carrying, and caring for our children. We also bring to light remarkable information from modern science that clearly tells us that experience and learning begin well before we take our first breath. The integration of these two different perspectives gives us the tools to ensure that our children are nourished by our thoughts, words, and actions. We are spiritual beings who have learned to manufacture physical forms. Although for the span of a lifetime we disguise ourselves as individual people, our essential nature remains that of unbounded consciousness . . . of pure potentiality . . . of Spirit. When you invite a soul into your life by conceiving a baby, you are assuming a sacred trust to love and nourish a divine impulse that is manifesting humanity. We are all expressions of that same unified field of existence, so creating a child is ultimately creating another statement of ourselves. The love and caring that we give to our children is an extension of the nurturing we give to ourselves. If we aim to create a nonviolent world, we must begin with love and nourishment in the womb.

Our world is complex and dynamic. At any one moment, we can point to situations and circumstance that give rise to great hope or great despair. There are regions on this planet where creativity, abundance, and spirituality are blooming and other spots where poverty, violence, and suffering are pervasive. Whatever the situation, we can be certain that all hope for the future resides in how we nurture our children. We have inherited everything we know from those who have preceded us and we have a choice as to what we pass along to the next generation. If we unconsciously perpetuate in our children the conflicts and misunderstandings that we inherited, we will have missed an opportunity to change the world. If, on the other hand, we expand our awareness to embrace compassion, unity, and love, we can genuinely reshape this world. The latter will ensure that our children will know themselves as the glorious, spiritual beings they are.

As loving parents, we all have one essential desire for our children: we wish for them to be happy. Recognizing this, we offer this guide to conscious parenting. We invite you to share our hope that all children will be blessed with *enchanted lives*—and we bring you this book in hopes of helping to create a healthier, more loving world.

Personalizing This Book

Every journey has the potential to take you beyond the limits of your mind to a deep place within your heart. As you travel through this book you will encounter many exercises designed to support your personal growth. Chapters include journaling, drawing, and visualization exercises designed to be playful opportunities for self-discovery. We believe that pregnancy can be a time of profound spiritual awakening as you listen deeply to the intuitive wisdom available in both your mind and body.

Journaling Your Pregnancy

When the mind is clear
You can see all the way
To the heart.

—STEVEN LEVINE

We suggest that you take some time every day of your pregnancy to jot down a few paragraphs about how you feel. Even on days when you believe you have nothing to say, take a few moments to write down your thoughts. Some women create a specific time each day to write, while others carry a journal with them, writing when they feel inspired. Let your journal be a truthful expression of your experiences. You might be inspired to draw pictures or doodle in your journal. Remain open to what comes to you.

Journaling will help you gain insights into your thoughts and feelings. Listening to your inner dialogue, you will connect to your baby and to deeper places inside you. Journaling can aid you in becoming more present in life. Far too often people look outside themselves to discover who they are, seeking out teachers, lectures, and workshops for the answers to the questions about how they are supposed to feel. Through journaling, you can tap into the flow of inner wisdom, insights, and answers that are accessible deep in your own being. As you attend to yourself in this way, you will be more conscious of your unborn baby's development and witness yourself blossoming as a parent.

Here's an example of a journal entry of a woman five months pregnant with her first child:

My Dear Angel,

You have been kicking and playing all day today inside my belly. Each kick brings my awareness to you. Throughout the day I close my eyes and give you all of my attention. I feel deeply connected to you already—it is hard to describe exactly how. It feels like I am thinking, imagining, feeling, connecting, and experiencing telepathy with you all in one. It is really an amazing feeling.

My belly is getting bigger each day. I love it when I look at my naked body in the mirror. Your dad looks at me in complete delight, which makes me feel sensual and womanly.

Your father is going to be such a great dad. You are going to love him. He drew a picture of you, himself, and me yesterday. We all have the biggest smiles and you are in the middle. Around us he wrote words describing all the different feelings we have had over the past few months. It describes the excitement of you coming and our worries about such a big change. It is a great picture. I am going to frame it and hang it in your room.

> I love you,
> Mom

Close your eyes and pay attention to how it feels to have a baby growing in your body. Become aware of your joys, concerns, and fears. Write them down without holding back. Don't worry about your spelling or grammar. Enjoy yourself! Light some incense or diffuse an aroma. Put on some favorite music. You may discover feelings that you haven't acknowledged before. Some of these feelings may even surprise you. Be open to and write about whatever comes to you.

Listening is a form of accepting.

—STELLA TERRILL MANN

Insight Through Drawing

Creating images and drawings to express your feelings and experiences can also be a powerful way to access your inner self. Pictures can bypass verbal language to directly reveal inner thoughts and emotions about your pregnancy, birth, and unborn baby. Although it is not uncommon for people to resist engaging in drawing, we encourage you simply to try the process. As a child you may have shut down drawing as a means for creative expression because you weren't as talented as you may have wanted to be, but drawing is an amazing avenue for personal growth. Give yourself permission not to be perfect. Allow your creativity to be expressed through your hands. Let yourself be wild and free. Find the childlike space inside you that loves to color and draw. Take out your crayons, chalk, paints, and clay. Release your inner critic and let yourself play. Obtain a journal or notebook to write and draw in. Find one that will allow you to be free and spontaneous. Keep some pens, colored pencils, and markers handy. As insights emerge and your creative forces flow, jot down the thoughts and images that come to mind.

Creative Imagination

When people's eyes are open
They see landscapes in the outer world.
When people's eyes are closed,
They see landscapes with their mind's eye.
People spend hours looking at outer landscapes,
But there is just as much to see
In inner landscapes.

—MICHAEL AND NANCY SAMUELS

Creative imagination is the process of invoking sensory experiences on the screen of your consciousness. Creative-imagination exercises offered throughout this book will enable you to connect deeply with your own body and your unborn baby. They can also help reduce stress during your pregnancy.

Each of us has inner experiences that are not visible from the outside; images, thoughts, and memories float through our awareness throughout the day. Although we usually refer to this process as visualization, any of the five senses may be involved. You may conjure up sounds, sensations, tastes, and smells in addition to visual images. When asked to remember your childhood home, for example, you might recall the shape of your piano, the soft texture of your favorite pillow, or the delicious flavors and fragrances of your mother's cooking. Entire scenes may come to life as you recall a particular circumstance or event. Your body and mind react to internal experiences much the way they react to external ones. Abundant psychological research demonstrates that your autonomic nervous system, which is responsible for regulating involuntary physiological functions, such as heart rate, blood pressure, hormone levels, and immune function, reacts to imaginary or recalled events just as if they were occurring in the actual world of forms and phenomena. If you vividly imagine relaxing at the beach, your body releases the same chemical messengers that are produced when you are actually enjoying a day at the shore. If you intensely recall an upsetting event, your heart rate, blood pressure, respiration, and metabolic processes respond as if you were encountering that stressful circumstance in real time. Using creative imagination, you can choose the happier event, accessing your inherent creative power to invoke healing, centering, and relaxation.

We believe in the power of imagination. Throughout this book we will invite you to exercise that talent, and like any skill, it will improve as you practice it. We may invite you to envision your baby growing inside your body or have you generate an image of how you'd like to see yourself in labor. Through creative imagination you will enhance your connection with your unborn baby long before she is in your arms. As you use your imagination, you will discover that you have the ability to create just about anything you want.

Pregnancy is a path that will take you beyond your mind and body. It will enliven your compassion and reveal the most intimate truths of your soul. This book is about discovering your heart and finding your path. Each step along the way is unique to you. Enjoy the journey.

We'll begin at the beginning of life—when two cells fuse and the spark that's generated ignites the fire of a new being.

CHAPTER 1

Creating a Baby

The body of a woman who is to conceive

Is being chosen as a channel

For the expression of divinity into materiality.

Although ovulation is a law of nature,

Conception is a law of God.

—EDGAR CAYCE

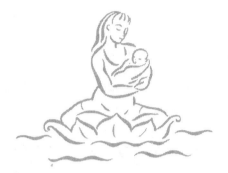

*W*hen does life begin? Some spiritual traditions see the origin of life as the moment a
soul intends to enter into human form.
Others see the beginning as a sparkle in the eye of a potential parent who wants to have a child. While biologists and
religious clergy may argue about whether or not life starts at
the moment of conception, convention has it that the day
a baby emerges from his mother's womb marks the beginning
of life. However you define life's origin, the sacred journey
of an egg and sperm merging to create a unique individual
is as marvelous and miraculous as the creation of the uni-

verse itself. Spirit and molecules intertwine to manifest a new life.

The blueprint for a human body is encoded in every cell of a human being, which contains forty-six chromosomes and more than thirty thousand genes. These genes, composed of DNA, provide blueprints for the proteins that ultimately form the chemicals, tissues, and organs of a person. They are responsible for the texture of your baby's hair, the color of his skin, and to some degree, the unique characteristics of his personality. With the unraveling of the human genome, we are closer than ever to understanding how DNA influences both physical and psychological traits, as well as our predisposition to illnesses. Still, we are a long way from fully unraveling the mystery of how a few genetic words can code for the unfathomable biological diversity on this planet.

In every human being, half of the forty-six chromosomes are contributed by the mother through her egg and half by the father through his sperm. The merging and reshuffling of the genetic potential of Mother with that of Father gives rise to the amazing variety of life. According to Ayurveda, these primordial cells, known as *shukra*, are the essence of biological intelligence, and the most important products of a living being.

When a young woman first begins menstruating, her ovaries contain tens of thousands of potential eggs. Each month, from the time menstruation begins until menopause, a number of her eggs begin the process of development, but usually just one fully ripens and is released. Over the course of a woman's reproductive years, only about four hundred eggs reach maturity and have the chance to develop into a human baby.

The egg or ovum is the largest cell in a woman's body and is about 100,000 times heavier than a sperm. It carries enough nourishment to sustain itself from the time it is released until it is implanted in the lining of the womb. This usually takes about five days, if along the way, the egg is fertilized.

Sperm cells, which carry the father's genetic material, are generated in a man's testes beginning in puberty and continuing throughout his life. Millions of new sperm cells are created each day, the vast majority of which are never released. During ejaculation, about three hundred million tiny sperm are released in a volume of about a teaspoon of seminal fluid. Only about three million sperm pass through the vagina into the uterus, most of which become lost or exhausted, so that less than three hundred enter into the fallopian tube where a ripe egg is waiting.

For sperm, the 12 inches from the cervix to the egg is longer than a marathon and takes about ten hours to navigate. In most cases, fertilization occurs shortly after an egg enters the fallopian tube on its way to the uterus. Sperm cells that choose the correct tube reach the egg, encircle it, and attach themselves to its outer layer. The final competitors release the powerful digestive enzymes contained in their caps, which carve microscopic openings through the egg's external coat. Only a single sperm is allowed to penetrate the egg, which then instantly closes its gates to all other contenders. The victorious sperm sheds its tail and head while its genes align with those of the egg. The runner-up sperm, with their heads in the outer layer of the egg, continue waving their tails. This has the effect of rotating the now fertilized egg, freeing it to move toward the womb. The egg and sperm, once comprising their individual energy and intelligence, entwine to embark on life's journey as a new entity—the seed of a unique human being.

Over the next four to six days, the fertilized egg floats down the fallopian tube. Along the way it divides several times, taking on the appearance of a mulberry. Some of the outer cells prepare to form the placenta, while the inner cells begin the differentiation process that ultimately results in your baby. By the time the little bundle reaches the uterus, the original fertilized egg cell, now known as a *blastocyst*, has already expanded to a collection of about a hundred cells.

While this multiplication is occurring, the inner lining of your womb prepares for implantation. Hormones produced by

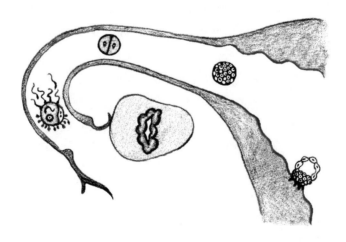

your ovary stimulate the glands and blood vessels of the inner uterus to become soft and succulent. When the blastocyst arrives, its outer layers are able to snuggle into the lush inner lining of the uterus. This begins the process of the embryonic baby tapping into Mother to nourish his body, mind, and soul. As many parents discover, it is not uncommon for this process to continue for decades to follow.

According to Ayurveda, an ember of consciousness is present in every living cell. As your new baby begins to take physical form, sparks of consciousness in the individual cells unite with each other, igniting self-awareness within the unborn child. This flame of awareness, known in Ayurveda as *Agni*, becomes brighter as the level of biological sophistication rises. The fire is fanned by the essential vital force, known as *Prana*, while the essence of biological integrity, *Ojas*, organizes the developing cells into a cohesive unified system. On a spiritual level these three primordial forces—Agni, Prana, and Ojas (or fire, breath, and earth)—are the essential building blocks of life. These elemental energies fuel one's brilliance, vitality, and love. The passion for life inherent in the soul of your baby begins to be expressed at the moment of conception, or perhaps, even before.

Why does life arise? According to Ayurveda, universal intelligence gives rise to life simply so it can evolve into complex expressions, capable of pondering and appreciating the mysteries of the universe. From this perspective, life is a cosmic masquerade, in which the goal is to uncover who is concealed. At the beginning of life, the disguise is quite transparent to the conscious mother who recognizes the deep spiritual connection that unites her baby's soul with her own. Her most important role from the moment of conception is to nurture her child so he can rediscover his essential spiritual nature.

In some traditions, this connection is believed to precede conception.

In certain African tribes, people believe that the spiritual birth of a child begins when his potential mother first imagines him. She goes to a silent place and listens for the baby's special song. When she hears it, she returns to her home and teaches it to her mate. While making love, they chant the song as an invitation for this soul to enter into their lives. Once pregnant, she regularly sings the song to her unborn baby and teaches it to the midwives in preparation for her birth. They sing the song while the woman is in labor and as the baby is born into the world. The child learns the theme song, which supports him through all the stages of his life. He uses his song to celebrate his moments of glory and comfort him in times of loss.

Growing a Baby

By the time the blastocyst finds its nest in the luxuriant lining of the womb, some of its cells are producing an important chemical called *human chorionic gonadotropin* or hCG. This substance stimulates the ovary to produce progesterone and estrogen, which nourish the womb until the placenta is able to make enough of these chemicals on its own. Levels of hCG are detectable in the blood of a pregnant woman as early as eight days after conception, and almost every pregnant woman has measurable levels by the eleventh day. Testing for this chemical is the basis of both urine and blood pregnancy tests. A level below 5 in the blood is considered negative, whereas a level above 25 is positive. HCG levels may rise to a peak of 250,000 between the eighth and tenth weeks and then gradually fall as you enter your second trimester of pregnancy.

We can only marvel at the intelligence that underlies the development of a complex human being from a cluster of apparently identical cells. Where are the laws written that govern this dance of life? They are written in the experiences of millions of years of evolutionary time. We can describe what happens, can set up the conditions by which it occurs through in vitro fertilization or cloning, but we cannot fully understand how each cell knows which genes to awaken and which are to be left dormant. We cannot explain how flawless mirror images of eyes, ears, arms, and legs are formed in perfect synchrony. We cannot explain how different parts of the nervous system "know" to reach out to each other across vast cellular distances to transmit critical information. The orchestration of life occurs from a deeper domain of existence, which is mysterious and incomprehensible. Every living being truly has a magical beginning.

Primordial Perception

Continuous cellular activity marks the first month of pregnancy, setting the stage for the development of your baby's tissues, organs, and physiological systems. As early as the fifth week after conception, the basic components of his nervous system are established, including a primitive brain, a spinal cord, and the sensory equipment for hearing, touching, seeing, tasting, and smelling. The anatomy needed to perceive and interpret the world forms rapidly once a new life comes into being.

HEARING IN THE WOMB

The acoustic system that enables your baby to hear develops through three different components—the outer ear, the middle ear, and the inner ear. The outer ear begins as little buds that gradually fuse to create your baby's sound-collecting dish. The middle ear is formed by linking up three tiny bones that transmit vibrations received by the outer ear to your baby's inner ear. The inner ear is a remarkable apparatus that translates the pitch and intensity of sound waves into specific electrical impulses, which then communicate this information to the hearing region of the brain. The equipment for your unborn baby to eavesdrop on the world is well developed by the time you enter your second trimester of pregnancy.

One of the earliest accounts of intrauterine hearing is described in the New Testament (Luke 1:44) when John's mother, Elizabeth, tells Mary, who is pregnant with Jesus, "The infant in my womb leaped for joy the moment I heard the voice of your greeting!" A number of modern studies have confirmed that by eighteen to twenty weeks of fetal life, your unborn child hears and responds to sounds in his environment. Although you might expect the womb to be a quiet place, it is actually quite rich in sounds and sensations. Tiny microphones placed within a pregnant uterus reveal that a multitude of audible vibrations enters your unborn baby's sanctum. Mother's heartbeat and digestive tract offer steady background noise, along with the pulsing rush of blood flowing through her major vessels.

The rhythm and pitch of human voices are clearly perceptible in the womb. An adult listening to conversations recorded through a miniature microphone placed in a womb can understand over half of the words spoken by a man and over a third of the words spoken by a woman standing in front of the pregnant woman. To your unborn baby, it is your voice that is most easily recognized. Unlike outside sounds, which are muffled to some degree, the voice of Mother is actually slightly amplified. If you are singing, the sound in your womb can reach more than 80 decibels, which is as loud as a ringing telephone or vacuum cleaner. Your fetus hears your voice both as an airborne sound and as vibrations that move directly through your organs, tissues, and bones. An unborn child becomes familiar with his mother's voice long before he emerges from the womb.

A baby learns to associate sounds in the womb with sensations of comfort or discomfort. The emotional state of his mother is communicated to the fetus through the molecules that she secretes. If Mother is engaged in a loving, nurturing conversation or listening to enjoyable music, her brain triggers the release of chemicals that reflect her calm, comfortable condition. These chemical messengers travel through the maternal and fetal circulations, now connected by the umbilical cord, entraining the unborn baby's feelings with those of Mother. If, on the other hand, Mother is involved in a heated argument, her body pulses with stress chemicals that can trigger discomfort in her fetus. It's easy to imagine the distress of an unborn baby regularly exposed to toxic sounds. His mother's heart races while her adrenal glands squirt out stress hormones. The unborn baby activates his own fight-or-flight response, but unfortunately can neither run from nor wrestle with the source of its provocation. The seeds of anxiety, apprehension, and hostility are sown in utero. The baby-to-be learns to associate sounds with inner sensations.

Do your best to avoid recurrent distressing sounds, since noise pollution has a negative effect on both Mother and Baby. Scientists report that mothers living along the flight path of a busy urban airport produce lower levels of growth-promoting hormones and are more likely to have smaller babies than those living an equal distance from the airport but not directly under the flight path. Similar findings have been reported in women who must work in factories where there is a constantly high noise level. To the extent that you can consciously choose, do your best to limit your exposure and that of your unborn baby to vibrations that distress.

On the other hand, it is not realistic to expect that you'll be able to completely avoid upsetting noises throughout your entire pregnancy. We are not suggesting you should worry about causing harm to your unborn baby anytime you get upset, have a disagreement, or listen to loud rock and roll music. Life inevitably brings loud moments that cannot nor necessarily should be avoided. We simply encourage you to be aware that the being inside of you is eavesdropping on your life. Whenever possible, expose yourself to nourishing rather than toxic sounds, knowing that whatever you are experiencing is simultaneously experienced by your unborn child.

FEELING IN THE WOMB

We feel our way in this world through two different interrelated systems. We have a *somesthetic* system that conveys information about touch, pressure, temperature, and pain, and we have a *vestibular* system that informs us how we are positioned in space. The basic anatomic architecture to perceive the world through the sense of touch is well formed by the time your unborn baby is about fifteen weeks old. A wide variety of sensory receptors develops in your baby's skin and joints, which tells his brain the texture, intensity, position, and temperature of anything he is touching or is touching him.

The vestibular or balance system helps us maintain the right position in relationship to our surroundings. Living on a planet with gravity requires us to know which way is up at all times. Although a human infant may not sit unsupported until six months of age, and it might be more than a year until he is standing and walking without help, the balance system required for these crucial functions is already developing by fourteen weeks of fetal life.

Babies in the womb respond to the sense of touch. During the fifth month a fetus can be seen touching his own face and sucking his thumb and fingers. Pressure through external massage leads to changes in fetal activity and heart rate, and by six months in the womb the unborn baby is as responsive to touch as a one-year-old baby. Unborn babies are also able to perceive changes in temperature and to feel pain. Injecting cold water into the amniotic fluid leads to withdrawal movements. If during an amniocentesis procedure the unborn baby is pricked with a needle, he reacts in ways suggesting he can perceive discomfort and does not appreciate the painful intrusion.

There is evidence that during the fifth month of fetal life your baby begins to orient himself in space. Studies have shown that unborn babies adjust themselves into more comfortable positions in the womb by kicking. The baby changes his position when the mother changes hers, and with abrupt maternal movements, sudden fetal motor responses and alterations in heart rate can be detected. These postural adjustments to normal maternal activity help the fetal navigation system develop in preparation for life outside the womb. Your own conscious movement through dance or yoga encourages healthy neuronal connections between the limbs, trunk, and brain of your growing baby.

Although we cannot say for certain that your unborn baby derives pleasure from your belly being massaged or stretching your back during yoga poses, we do know that when you are feeling comfortable, your fetus is bathed in the comforting chemicals that your body produces. Moving with awareness benefits both you and your unborn baby.

SEEING IN THE WOMB

The womb is a pretty dark place, yet some light does filter through. The earliest evidence of a visual system appears by one month of gestation, and by the end of the first trimester, your unborn baby's eyes have all their essential components. The visual system continues to develop in complexity throughout pregnancy and beyond, since an infant's ability to process visual information is not complete until several months after birth.

The eyelids of a fetus begin to open at about twenty weeks of gestation, and there is pretty good evidence that between 2 percent and 10 percent of visual outside light is able to reach the rudimentary eyes of a fetus. When bright lights are shined onto a pregnant woman's belly, the unborn baby will show an increase in motor activity and acceleration in heart rate. An indirect but more important role of visual stimulation on your unborn child is played by what you are looking at. Violent images served up by the media stimulate your body's stress response, which is communicated to your baby. Beautiful, pleasing images create physiological changes that are rejuvenating and balancing. Again, we are not suggesting that you walk around with blinders on but do encourage you to get a dose of nourishing images on a regular basis.

TASTING IN THE WOMB

Your baby's taste buds are present as early as twelve weeks of fetal life and are well developed by early in the second trimester. They are initially found throughout his mouth, but eventually become concentrated on his tongue and palate. Taste buds are connected to nerve fibers by the twelfth week and are functioning by the fifteenth week.

Studies have suggested that an unborn baby will increase or decrease his swallowing based upon the flavors present in the amniotic fluid, and it looks as though even unborn babies like sweets. Intrauterine studies have shown that if sweetened solutions are introduced into the amniotic fluid, babies swallow more, whereas when bitter substances are injected, babies swallow less. Your unborn child also has the ability to distinguish sour and salty flavors. From very early on we have the ability to distinguish good-tasting substances from bad ones.

As we'll explore later in this book, the best way to ensure that you are receiving optimal nourishment is to be certain that your diet includes the six primary tastes on a daily basis. Your unborn child is not only nourished by what you eat, but may actually be capable of tasting what you taste.

SMELLING IN THE WOMB

As adults, we perceive the fragrance of the world through tiny specialized receptors in our nasal passages that sample the air for odor-rich molecules. The cellular apparatus for perceiving aromas appears as early as the fourth week of fetal life and is well developed by halfway through pregnancy. The obvious question is, "Is there anything for your baby to smell?" and the answer is yes. Amniotic fluid naturally contains a large assortment of fragrant substances, which vary from day to day depending upon what you ingest. Premature babies react to a variety of scents, and fetal mammals of many species respond to aromatic chemicals infused into amniotic fluid. Certain spices such as curry and garlic seep into the amniotic fluid, and at birth some babies will smell like a spice from food the mother has eaten the night before.

Babies remember smells and tastes they are exposed to in the womb. Studies have shown that newborn mammals, from rodents to humans, show preferences for substances with fragrances they experienced before birth. Baby rats prefer beverages containing apple juice if they were exposed to the flavor of apples while in the womb. Newborn human infants favor the smell of their own amniotic fluid for several days after birth. After birth, if a newborn baby is given the choice of suckling on her mother's unwashed breast, which secretes a smell similar to the smell of amniotic fluid, or on a breast that has been washed, more than 75 percent of the time the newborn will choose the breast with the familiar amniotic smell. As is true for all the other senses, your olfactory experiences during pregnancy become your baby's experiences. As we'll explore in detail in Chapter 2, you can use this understanding to enhance both your baby's and your own well-being.

The Gifts of Pregnancy

Pregnancy is a precious opportunity to be mindful and reflective. With awareness you can tune into your inner state, becoming more conscious to yourself, to your unborn baby, and to each moment of your life. Take time to sit and listen deeply, and you will begin to notice the subtle ways you and your unborn child react to the choices you are making. By tuning into your own sensory experiences, you will find yourself slowing down naturally and becoming more present. You will gain clarity in your life and experience more inner peace. This will have a profound impact on your unborn baby's first experiences of the world.

Exercise

Sit or lie down, and allow your eyes to close. Taking in a few slow, deep breaths, bring awareness into your body. Look around inside. Feel and envision the space. Notice the shades, subtle colors, and textures within you. Feel your breath as it moves through you. Sense its vibration and begin to listen to its sound. For the next several breaths follow the sound. Let it take you deeper inside yourself. Feel your heartbeat and the pulsation of life within you. With each in-breath, allow the tenderness of your heart to surround your baby. With each out-breath, create an image of your baby growing inside your body. Breathe in tenderness; breathe out a clearer vision of your baby. Own your part in creating this little being. Breathe in joy for the miracle occurring in your body; as you breathe out, feel your love for this new being developing within you.

The Journey into Life

We've been emphasizing the development of your baby's sensory systems, because it's so important to change our notion of unborn children from being isolated, unresponsive clusters of cells to primordial sentient beings influenced by the sounds, sensations, sights, tastes, and smells in their environment. Since your baby has limited ability to influence his experiences, it becomes your responsibility to choose those that provide maximal nourishment and minimal toxicity. Your choices provide the raw materials that enable your baby's soul to create its body, senses, and mind.

The sequential development of your baby's body is an expression of nature's synchronous intelligence. The development of the right side of the body does not trigger the development of the left side; rather, the simultaneous emergence of symmetrical components is orchestrated by an underlying intelligence. This intelligence is beyond cause and effect, beyond time and space, and beyond beginnings and endings. Whether you call this force nature, spirit, or

God, its ability to bring forth form out of formlessness is magical and miraculous.

Let's review some milestones that mark this extraordinary journey from a fertilized egg to a complete newborn human being:

Days 1 to 14 The time between the first day of your last menstrual period and the day of ovulation.

End of week 2 Father's sperm fertilizes mother's egg in the fallopian tube.

Week 3 The fertilized egg divides several times and implants in the lining of the uterus.

Week 4 The embryo differentiates into three different layers:

> An *outer layer*—destined to become your baby's skin, nervous system, hair, and nails
>
> A *middle layer*—destined to become your baby's muscles, bones, heart, and blood vessels
>
> An *inner layer*—destined to become your baby's digestive tract and urinary system

The embryo receives nourishment and oxygen from the placenta through the umbilical cord. Everything the embryo and fetus require until birth will travel back and forth through this cord. The placenta, although capable of filtering many substances from your body, is not able to filter them all. Many drugs and toxins can still pass through the placental barrier and enter your baby's body.

Week 6 Your baby's primitive heart is beating, although the embryo is less than ¼ inch long. Primitive eyes, arms, and legs are present.

Week 8 The embryo now becomes known as a fetus, which in Latin means "young one." He weighs less than half an ounce. The digestive tract is forming and blood is carrying oxygen and nourishment to cells through his primitive circulatory system.

Week 10 The fetus is about 1 inch long, with recognizable eyes, ears, fingers, and toes. Internal organs are functioning, and his brain is growing at an incredible rate of 250,000 new cells every minute!

Week 12 Your unborn baby's face looks very human, with a tiny nose and chin. He is over 3 inches long and weighs about 2 ounces. The fetus can flex and extend his fingers. Sexual differentiation is now apparent.

Week 16 Fine hair (lanugo) is developing on his head. Your baby is actively moving and making sucking motions with his mouth. His bones are becoming harder and muscles are developing.

Week 20 Tiny nails appear on your baby's fingers and toes. His entire body is covered with fine hair. Mother can feel fetal movements, called quickening. The fetal heartbeat can be heard with a stethoscope. Your baby is about 8 inches in length.

Week 24 Your baby now weighs over 1 pound, and is just under a foot in length. His eyebrows and eyelashes are well formed. The fine air sacs in the lungs are almost functional.

Week 28 Although immature, your baby's lungs are developed to the point that survival is possible outside the womb. His eyelids open and close. His weight is over $2\frac{1}{2}$ pounds and he may be 15 inches long.

Week 32 Your baby's bones are well developed but still soft. Rhythmic breathing movements are present. The nervous system is steadily developing and your baby is learning to regulate his body temperature. Body fat is accumulating.

Week 36 The fetus is between 16 and 19 inches long and weighs about 6 pounds. If born prematurely at this stage, there is a high likelihood of survival.

Weeks 38 to 40 Your baby is considered full term, and is ready to begin his life outside of the womb.

The Miracle of Creation

Nature creates within you an entire person complete with all his parts in just forty weeks. Throughout pregnancy your body is your unborn baby's universe. You are the rivers, sunlight, earth, atmosphere, and sky for this being growing within you. Your baby's body, mind, and soul are intimately intertwined with your own. Together you express the creative flow of life.

In each moment, your unborn baby is immersed in the

sounds and vibrations of your heartbeat and breath. He feels your stress, tension, and fear along with your joy, happiness, and peace. Whenever you move, laugh, cry, eat, eliminate, or rest, your unborn baby responds. The potential of your child's life is encoded in each of his cells, while the environment of your body can either nurture or disturb this growth. Accept this responsibility with joy, for each healthy choice that you make on behalf of your unborn baby nourishes you as well. Your pregnancy can be a magical beginning for both you and your baby.

Exercise

Sit comfortably and allow your eyes to close. Feel yourself gently inhaling and exhaling. Allow your awareness to be inside your body. As you inhale, feel the nourishment and oxygen that you bring in, from the universe, from the source. As you feel this air filling your body, notice how it moves into your soft belly. Feel how it encircles your baby. Receive the sensations and nourishment in each breath. Now exhale and release this air, allowing it to flow back out into the universe. Continue breathing like this for the next few minutes. Breathe in, filling your belly; breathe out, releasing to the universe—each breath nourishing you and your baby.

Now bring your awareness to the space around your womb. Imagine yourself drifting through your uterine wall and amniotic sac and begin to feel yourself floating inside your womb. Imagine submerging deeper into the amniotic fluid and feel yourself floating here with your baby. Feel how soft and silky this fluid is and notice that it is just the right temperature for your baby. As your eyes wander through the space and semidarkness inside your womb—take in a breath—feel what it is like to be inside your body. These are the sensations your baby is experiencing as he grows inside you.

Look around the inner surfaces of your womb and find where the placenta is attached to your uterine wall. Take a moment to honor this organ that is continuously nourishing your baby. Feel how it is helping to keep him alive. As you continue to look around, see if you can find the umbilical cord, which is attached to the placenta. This is your baby's lifeline. Let your awareness flow down along this cord until you can see where it is connected to your baby's belly. See your baby here now—alive and growing inside your body. Feel yourself right here next to him. Take a few moments to feel this amazing little being—who is metamorphosing inside your belly. Feel how incredible it is to have a little person transforming and growing inside you. You are the entire universe for your baby. Experience yourself as his mother—notice how you are protecting him as he develops and grows. Look at his little body. See his fingers and his toes, his arms and legs, his tiny torso and head. Take a few moments to gaze at his face—and imagine what it will be like to look into his eyes for the first time. Imagine how it will feel to hold him in your arms. Become aware of your body holding him right now inside the warm nest of your womb.

Whenever you feel ready, gently bring your awareness

back to your breath. Feel your breath moving in and out of your body. Notice your belly rising and falling with each breath. Become aware of the sensation of the air in the room floating around you. Begin to move your body any way that feels good. As you feel ready, slowly open your eyes.

Take a few minutes to note in your journal how it feels to have a baby growing inside your body. See if you can conjure up a picture of your baby and take some time to draw this image.

Enliven Through Your Attention

• Place your hands on your belly a few times throughout the day and send loving thoughts to your unborn baby.

• Journal each day about your experiences.

• Early in your pregnancy, plant a tree or flowering bush to symbolize the growth of your baby in the womb. After your baby is born, you can take care of the plant together.

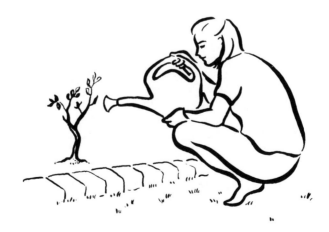

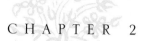

CHAPTER 2

Womb Ecology

Oh mighty one, the ancient inscrutable,

without name or form,

Disguised as Brahman, Abraham, the Primordial One,

You come to us as the gift of a child.

Salutations, salutations to you a million times,

For manifesting Yourself in every grain of creation.

—DEEPAK CHOPRA

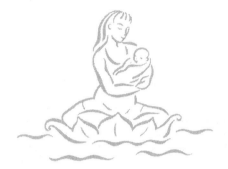

*T*here is an expression in Ayurveda that says, "What you see you become." In the West we have the phrase, "You are what you eat." Although these sayings come from different cultures, they are, in essence, both saying the same thing. Our experiences shape us. Whether you are hearing, feeling, seeing, tasting, or smelling, your experiences in each moment mold who you are. Your body and mind are created from your accumulated experiences.

Ayurveda suggests that if you want to understand your past, examine your body now. We can carry that further. If you wish to predict what your body will be like in the future, consider your experiences now. Each impulse of experience is being metabolized into the molecules of your body. Although it may be obvious that the food you eat becomes the matter of your body, it is equally true that the sounds you hear, the sensations you feel, the sights you see, and the aromas you smell are transformed into the physical molecules that make up your body. Your body is a field of living information and intelligence.

In recent years neurobiologists have provided us scientific explanations for this process. Through advanced technology, including brain-mapping studies and positron-emission tomography (PET) scans, we now know that every sensory perception and its associated emotional reaction leads to changes in the electricity and chemistry of your physiology. Your sensory experiences have either life-supporting or life-damaging effects on your mind and body. Even imaginary experiences can have potent physiological effects. Try this simple exercise:

Imagine hearing a shrieking ambulance go by.

Imagine listening to a Bach violin concerto.

Imagine being stung by a bee.

Imagine holding a baby in your arms.

Imagine witnessing an automobile accident.

Imagine watching a dramatic sunset.

Imagine tasting a bitter medicine.

Imagine biting into a juicy, sweet mango.

Imagine the smell of a skunk.

Imagine the aroma of a Hawaiian flower.

Each of these sensations, pleasurable or uncomfortable, imaginary or real, changes your body. When sensory stimulation is soothing, your body releases health-promoting chemicals. When it is toxic or negative, stress hormones are released. These various chemicals have the ability to nourish or deplete your body. Your nervous system plays a key role in this process. It is an amazing apparatus that identifies, filters, interprets, and responds to the energy and information you receive through your senses. When you hear the howl of a newborn baby, your brain processes the raw sensory data, labels it as a cry, interprets it as a statement of distress, and activates a response. These neurophysiological changes affect every cell of your being. Your interpretations, emotions, and feelings are encoded into chemical messengers that filter through your body.

Your thoughts and words are literally made into flesh. When you feel stressed, you release chemicals coded for stress, and every cell in your body receives the message. When you feel joyful, your body produces natural pleasure chemicals called endorphins and encephalins. When you are peaceful and relaxed, you release chemicals similar to prescription tranquilizers. Your body is an expression of your experiences.

Throughout pregnancy your unborn baby's cells are also being informed of your experiences and your sensations. As we discussed in the last chapter, the environment in your womb is rich with sounds and sensations, and your impressions of the world continually filter through to your baby. Your unborn child is a resilient and adaptable little being,

more aware, responsive, and interactive with her environment than scientists previously imagined. In the absence of
too much stress from your body, your baby's nervous system
works smoothly. When you're calm and centered, your baby
is able to grow peacefully, in tune with her own biological
rhythms.

Adrenaline, noradrenaline, oxytocin, serotonin, and most
other messenger molecules are transported across the placenta and influence your unborn baby. These chemicals generate a cascade of responses in your body, and in the body of
your unborn child.

Studies using ultrasound monitoring have shown that
within moments after a pregnant woman experiences a stressful event that generates anxiety, her unborn baby responds by
accelerating her heart rate or kicking strongly.

Awareness is the key factor in helping you create a nurturing environment for your baby. Rather than running on
automatic pilot, use the opportunity provided by your pregnancy to become mindful of your environment and the
effects it has on you and your baby. Learn to nurture yourself
by seeking out experiences that are nourishing and avoiding
those that are toxic. You can do so by consciously promoting
balance in your body through each of your five senses.

Exercise

Stop for a moment and focus on the sights around you.
Notice the colors, the size, and the shapes of objects within

your environment. Observe the textures of each object you perceive. Close your eyes and become aware of the sounds surrounding you right now. Listen deeply to each one. Become aware of the sensations of touch that are stimulating your skin at this moment. Feel the clothing on your body and the pressure of your feet against the ground. Gently stroke your arm and notice the sensations that your touch creates in your body. Take a deep breath and smell the aromas in the air. Lick your lips and taste the flavors and sensations in your mouth. Notice how by paying attention you have enlivened each of your five senses.

Awakening Your Inner Pharmacy Through the Five Windows to Your Soul

In ancient India a senior class of Ayurvedic medical students was given a final assignment to find things that had no therapeutic value. Only one student, Jivaka, returned empty-handed, saying that anything he put his attention on influenced his mind and body. The sounds of birds singing, the sensations of the breeze on his face, watching the sunset, tasting an herb, smelling a fragrant flower—each of these experiences had a therapeutic effect on him and, therefore, could be considered a form of medicine. Jivaka was declared valedictorian of his class and went on to become the personal physician to the Buddha.

Nourish Your Baby and Yourself Through Sound

The sounds that surround you play an important role in balancing your biological rhythms. Nourishing sounds are as important to your health as nourishing food. The German philosopher Martin Heidegger said, "Thinking is a subtle form of hearing." We hear the thoughts we think, and when they are powerful enough, we feel them as well. Thoughts that we feel are called emotions. Think of the word *mother*. First you hear the thought as a sound. Then, almost immediately, you'll find that you can feel the emotion that the word *mother* generates inside you. Now if you close your eyes and imagine the word *mother* again, you will be able to conjure up an image associated with the word *mother* in your mind. Sounds have the ability to bring forth sensations from all five of your senses. Think of the word *lemon*. As you conjure up the sour fruit in your awareness, you may begin to salivate as the word evokes the object it names. Thought becomes form, the word is made flesh.

Make a commitment to provide your unborn baby with a healthy dose of nourishing sounds on a regular basis. Take time to listen to music that inspires you. Although the significance of the "Mozart effect," which suggests that listening to classical music would make your baby more intelligent, is debatable, there is plenty of information that supports the view that music can soothe your body, mind, and soul. Studies have shown that listening to pleasing sounds can lower blood pressure, enhance immunity, and reduce anxiety.

Create your own cache of musical remedies. According to Ayurveda, there are three primary ways you can lose balance. First, excessive turbulence in your mind can lead to anxiety and insomnia. This is known as a *Vata*, or Wind, imbalance. Second, you can become overheated with feelings of irritation, frustration, and anger. This is referred to as a *Pitta*, or Fire, imbalance. Finally, you can become sluggish and stagnant, resulting in lethargy and fatigue, known in Ayurveda as a *Kapha*, or Earth, imbalance. You can use music to balance any of these situations. If you are feeling anxious or having trouble sleeping at night due to a turbulent mind, listen to music that is gentle and calming. If you are feeling irritable and ill-tempered, introduce music that is soothing and cooling. If you are feeling congested and listless, try listening to music that is invigorating and revitalizing. Play these sounds when you're relaxing, taking a bath, or getting massaged. Listening to your favorite selections at other times will trigger the memory of these relaxing experiences, which will be of benefit to you throughout your pregnancy and during labor. Some of our favorite musical selections are suggested below.

The sounds of nature also have a balancing effect on your mind and body and can help reconnect you to your essential state of peacefulness. Go for walks where you are exposed to those sounds that remind you of the timeless intelligence that underlies all of creation, including the creation of your unborn child. Pay attention to the breezes rustling the leaves, the ocean waves lapping up against the shore, the rushing of water in a stream, a waterfall cascading in the woods, and the songs of birds warbling on a warm summer day. Take time to listen to the natural vibrations that surround you.

Play an active role in your unborn child's acoustic experience, making a conscious commitment to choose nurturing auditory stimuli for you and your fetus. Ask your husband or partner to participate in the process. Have him read poetry or tell stories to you and your baby-to-be. Studies have shown that newborn babies, whose fathers spoke to them while in the womb, respond to their dad's soothing voice within the first few hours after birth.

The unborn baby begins to show behavioral responses to outside sound at about sixteen weeks and appears to be listening much of the day by twenty-four weeks, when the structures of the ear are fully formed.

Create a nickname or term of endearment for your unborn child and speak to her often. Recite love poems, read inspiring stories, and sing lullabies to your baby. Try listening to sounds that traditionally have been used to rejoice in spirit, such as Gregorian, Vedic, Hebrew, Native American, Celtic, or Hawaiian chants.

Remind yourself on a daily basis to stop and listen to the sounds in your environment and notice how you feel. Your unborn baby is also interacting, both directly and indirectly, with the sounds around you. When you generate coherence and comfort in your body through sound, you create a loving and nurturing environment for your unborn baby.

Suggested Music During Pregnancy

VATA

CALMING, RELAXING

Magic of Healing — Vata	Bruce & Brian Becvar
Angel Love	Aeoliah
Collaborations into the Moment	Steven Halpren & Master Charles
Om Mani Padme Hum	Master Charles

PITTA

SOOTHING, COOLING

Magic of Healing — Pitta	Bruce & Brian Becvar
Inner Flute	Flute for the Spirit
Bamboo Waterfall	Wind Chimes and Bells
Waterworks	Enya

KAPHA

INVIGORATING, ENERGIZING

Magic of Healing — Kapha	Bruce & Brian Becvar
The Essence	Deva Premal
Live on Earth	Krishna Das
The Rising	Bruce Springsteen

The soothing sound of your voice can have a profoundly nourishing influence on her. She loves to listen to the voice of your partner as well. At birth your baby will recognize both your voices.

Nurture Your Baby and Yourself Through Touch

The skin is your largest sense organ and it is rich with health-promoting potential. Its surface contains thousands of nerve receptors that transmit healing impulses to your body and mind. Through the sensations of touch you can use your skin to access this healing benefit for you and your unborn baby. Touch releases chemicals that have relaxing and health-promoting effects. When you are gently stroked or therapeutically touched, your stress level declines, your circulation improves, and your body's natural pleasure-enhancing molecules are enlivened. These health-promoting chemicals travel through both the maternal and fetal circulations. Massage also improves immune function, reducing Mother's susceptibility to colds and flu. A massage feels wonderful whether or not you are pregnant. When you are feeling comfortable and relaxed, your unborn child also benefits. As you relax, you may find that your baby enjoys the feeling so much that she begins to move and kick playfully, while at other times you may feel her contentedly resting.

Studies have shown that pregnant women who receive

massage sleep better and have lower levels of anxiety and depression. Massaged mothers experience fewer complications during labor and have a lower incidence of premature deliveries. There is also evidence that infants born of mothers who have received massages regularly during pregnancy have fewer problems during the first few weeks after birth.

Exercise

Several times during the day, tenderly place your hands on your belly. Imagine yourself holding your baby as she sleeps or kicks inside your womb. Gently massage your belly while speaking softly to her. Connect with your baby through the sense of touch, even before she is in your arms.

Nurturing Through Touch

Seek out nurturing touch throughout your pregnancy, from your husband or partner, from your family members and friends. Find a professional massage therapist who has experience with pregnant women. You can also gain many of the healing and soothing benefits of touch by performing an oil massage on yourself each day. According to Ayurveda, a daily self-massage is one of the most balancing components of a health-promoting daily routine. Try the following procedure before or after your daily bath or shower. If you are having trouble sleeping, perform the oil massage before bed, followed by a warm aromatherapy bath. Be sure to perform the massage over a towel or mat so that you do not slip and always remove the oil from your feet before moving around.

The subtle effects of different massage oils can be used to balance your mind and body. Oils that are considered warmer and heavier, such as sesame, walnut, and almond, are helpful in pacifying mental turbulence due to a Vata imbalance. Cooler oils, such as coconut, olive, and avocado, are helpful in soothing irritability related to a Pitta imbalance. Lighter oils, including sunflower, safflower, and mustard seed, help improve circulation and relieve the congestion associated with a Kapha imbalance. All-natural vegetable, nut, or seed oils nourish and soothe the tissues.

The style and intensity of the massage strokes also influence the effects of the massage. If you are feeling anxious or having trouble sleeping, use a firm, grounding massage stroke. If you are feeling overheated or irritable, use a gentler stroke. If you are feeling congested or bloated, try a deeper, more vigorous stroke. Listen to the needs of your body, and stay present in the process.

SELF-MASSAGE (USUALLY PERFORMED OVER FIVE TO TEN MINUTES)

Begin by warming the oil under hot water. Pour a small amount of oil in your hands and use it to massage your scalp vigorously. Cover your entire scalp with small, circular strokes as if you were shampooing your hair. As your fingers caress your scalp, close your eyes and enjoy the sensations.

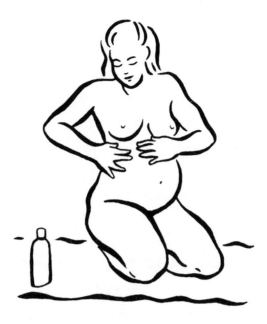

Next move to your face and ears. Gently massage the backs of your ears. According to both Ayurveda and traditional Chinese medicine, your ears have many sensitive nerve endings that connect to all areas of your body, so massaging them is especially calming. Apply a little more oil to your hands and with circular motions, stroke your temples, forehead, eyebrows, nose, cheeks, jaw, mouth, and chin. Massage the front, back, and sides of your neck.

Next massage your arms. The process for both your upper and lower limbs is to use a circular motion over the joints and a back-and-forth motion over the long bones. Apply the oil in a circular motion to your shoulders, back and forth on your upper arms, circular at the elbows, back and forth over the forearms, circular at the wrists, and then massage each finger from the base of your palm to the fingertip.

Be very gentle over your trunk. Use large circular motions over your breasts, belly, and lower abdomen. As you massage your belly and pass your hands over your womb, send love and tenderness to your growing baby. Apply a little more oil and reach around to massage your back as best as you can. Ask your partner to massage any areas you can't reach on your own.

Finish with your legs and feet. Massage your legs as you did your arms, using circular motions at your hips, back-and-forth motions over your thighs, circular over the knees, and long back-and-forth strokes on your lower legs. Very gently apply circular motions over the ankles, and then vigorously massage your feet with a back-and-forth motion and then stroke and pull each toe.

If possible, allow the oil to soak into your body. Leaving on a thin layer of oil will protect and nourish your skin and help keep your muscles warm throughout the day. If you take a shower after the massage, wash with mild soap.

MINIMASSAGE (ONE TO TWO MINUTES)

If you don't have time for a full-body massage, a short one is better than none at all. Your head and feet are the most important parts of your body to cover, and this can be accomplished in a very short time.

Rub some warm oil into your scalp, using the small, circular motions described above. Use your palm to massage your forehead from side to side.

Gently massage your temples, using circular motions. Then gently rub the outside of your ears. Spend a few moments massaging the back and front of your neck. With a little more oil, massage both feet with the flat of your hand. Work the oil around your toes with your fingertips, and then vigorously massage the soles of your feet with brisk back-and-forth motions of your palms. Sit quietly for a few seconds to relax and let the oil soak in, and then bathe as usual.

MASSAGING THE PERINEUM

The perineum refers to the structures around the floor of the pelvis, covering the area from the pubic bone in front to the coccyx bone at the tip of your spine. Although the soft tissues around the perineum become elastic and stretchy during birth, we recommend you begin tenderly massaging your perineal area with oil about four to six weeks before your due date to help prepare for delivery. This may help reduce the

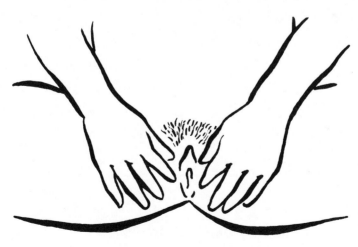

likelihood of tearing or injury and can facilitate the healing of tissues after birth. It will also help to familiarize you with the feeling of your perineum stretching.

Nourish Your Baby and Yourself Through Sight

You are your baby's window to the world. Everything that you see influences your body and your unborn child. When you gaze lovingly into the eyes of your partner and become filled with comforting feelings, you communicate your sensations to your baby. When you laugh joyfully at children playing or witness a dazzling sunset, something shifts inside you. Studies have shown that visual experiences evoke chemical responses throughout the body that can uplift or depress us. When medical students were shown videos with violent scenes, they experienced suppression of their immune system, whereas when they watched images of compassionate acts, their immune function was enhanced. You can change your body's chemistry by paying attention to what you see. To the extent possible, limit your exposure to visual experiences that upset you, such as scary or violent movies and disturbing television shows. Seek out visual experiences that delight you.

Upon awakening in the morning, become aware of the first things you see when you look around. Notice whether or not your day's first sights are pleasing to your eyes.

Throughout the day remain conscious of the images you see. Become aware of how they affect you. Before going to bed, gaze into the sky, taking in the experience of the stars, the moon, and the whole galaxy. Tune into the sensations that are created in your body as you take in these sights. Close your eyes and notice how you feel. Breathe into the feelings.

Search for visual experiences that uplift you. Walk through gardens and spend time at the beach. Make a point of getting outside each day. As you move through nature, enjoy the sights of the luxuriant plants and magnificent trees in your environment, absorbing the oxygen they are releasing to you. Observe the colors, textures, and shapes of everything you see. People, things, and events "out there" all become a part of who we are "in here."

By the time the fetus is thirteen weeks old, her eyes are well developed. Her eyelids will now close until the seventh month of life when the eyelids unseal again.

Human beings are visual creatures, and our interpretation of what we see strongly influences our sense of comfort or discomfort. Although while in the womb your baby's experiences are limited, there is evidence that shortly after birth, a newborn is able to recognize and process visual information.

A fascinating study dating back to the 1970s by researcher T. G. R. Bower showed that even at a few hours old, newborns preferred looking at their mother's face over another woman's. To perform this study, pairs of female faces were flashed on a video screen in front of infants, who were given pacifiers to suck. If a newborn baby sucked one way, an unfamiliar woman would appear. If she sucked another way, her mother would appear. After a period of watching and sucking, the newborns tended more often to suck in the way that brought their own mother's face onto the screen. One wonders if a baby begins to imagine her mother's face based upon the sounds and sensations he hears in the womb, in the same way that you as an adult might imagine what a person looks like when you are speaking to them on the telephone, or when you hear someone on the radio. We create pictures from the sounds we hear, and your unborn baby may be doing the same. For many reasons, when you have a choice, choose to see things that you would want your baby to see, and reduce your exposure to visual images from which you would want to protect your baby. This will add to your well-being as well as to your baby's.

Nourish Your Baby and Yourself Through Taste

We have a natural tendency to sample the world by putting things into our mouths. Infant children experience this inclination when they go through the oral phase. During this stage, parents quickly learn to clear their homes of objects that can be placed into the mouths of their young ones, because there is this intrinsic impulse to taste things. Over millions of years of evolutionary time, human beings have used this tendency to identify food sources that sustain and nourish us.

The sense of taste assesses the nourishing potential of everything that passes through your mouth. Taste provides clues as to whether or not a food will add to or detract from feelings of well-being. If a potential food source has a palatable flavor, this indicates to the brain that taking more of it is beneficial. If it has an offensive taste, the message is to leave it alone. In this way, people in every culture around the world have identified nurturing foods that became essential components of their diet.

Aside from breathing, eating is our most important bodily function. Your taste buds have exquisitely sensitive receptors that take part in your body's ability to convert food into energy.

People often overthink their nutrition. They try to balance their diets according to the latest recommendations by nutritional experts who advocate varying proportions of carbohydrates, proteins, and fats. From the standpoint of Ayurveda, nutrition need not be complicated; nature has encoded the intelligence of food into packets that provide the energy and information required to create and maintain a healthy body. This area is a vitally important part of a healthy pregnancy, so we will devote the entire next chapter to nourishing you and your baby.

Nourish Your Baby and Yourself Through Smell

Smell is one of your most primal senses and is intimately associated with memory and emotion. The aroma of cookies baking in the oven or the scent of lilac bushes in a park may evoke images, memories, and emotions from your past. Although you might not always be aware of it, your brain is very sensitive to the fragrance-carrying molecules in the air around you. Aromas provide information about your environment and subtly influence your moods, behavior, and energy levels.

The brain is designed to process and respond to olfactory information through the limbic system. This circuitry coordinates the basic physiological functions responsible for regulating your appetite, sexual desire, blood pressure, heartbeat, sleep cycles, memory, and emotions. Your sense of smell plays a role in these critical functions because in most higher animal species, olfaction is used to determine sources of nourishing food, partners suitable for mating, the boundaries of territory, and the presence of enemies. Although human beings are less tuned into their sense of smell than many other animals, we still respond to odors and scents in primitive and powerful ways.

Each day you take the world in through your sense of smell.

Close your eyes for a moment and see if you can conjure up the different scents that surrounded you today. You may recall some that were pleasing and find others that were offensive. As you evoke them, see if you can sense how you felt as a result of your exposure to them. Pleasant aromas soothe your being and unpleasant odors may annoy or deplete you.

During pregnancy, you can take advantage of your sense of smell by consciously choosing aromas that are balancing and nourishing. There are two basic ways to consciously use aromas to enhance a state of well-being. The first is to link a pleasing fragrance to a positive experience. When you are practicing meditation, relaxing in a yoga pose, listening to soothing music, or receiving a massage, diffuse a calming aroma such as lavender, geranium, or juniper in the room. Your brain will begin to associate the smell with the experience, so that at other times, just inhaling the aroma will help you relax.

The second way to benefit from smell is by taking advantage of the specific therapeutic properties of essential oils. These oils are extracted

The earliest components of the olfactory system appear by six weeks of fetal age. Although it is not possible to assess exactly how soon and how well a fetus can perceive smells, we do know that immediately after birth, an infant is capable of identifying familiar odors and scents.

from the roots and stems of flowers, fruits, herbs, and trees and have direct effects on the nervous system. Essential oils, which are sometimes known as the soul of a plant, have a long-established role in healing systems around the world. In Ayurveda, fragrances are used for their medicinal and spiritual properties. We recommend that you keep a small vial of an essential oil with you, so it is available to you whenever you could benefit from its specific therapeutic characteristics.

Listed below are essential oils that can be used to calm, soothe, or invigorate your mind-body system and are safe to use during pregnancy.

Essential Oils

OIL	SPECIAL EFFECTS
CALMING AND GROUNDING	
Chamomile	Balances digestion
Geranium	Mood elevating
Lavender	Pain relieving
Vanilla	Helps induce sleep
SOOTHING AND COOLING	
Jasmine	Mood elevating, anti-inflammatory
Neroli	Balances digestion, refreshing
Patchouli	Grounding, skin replenishing
Mandarin	Calming, soothing to nervous system

Cinnamon	Stimulating, helps reduce digestive gas
Ginger	Digestive stimulant, anti-nausea
Juniper	Clears the mind, restores confidence
Clary Sage	Decongesting and detoxifying

Exercise

Choose one of the essential oils above that is soothing to you. Create a comfortable place to lie down where you can relax, or take a warm bath. Begin diffusing the essential into the air or pour a few drops into your tub.

Once you are comfortable, allow your eyes to close and begin to feel your breath. Notice the sensations in your body. Feel yourself breathing into your belly and notice the scent of your aroma encircling you. Breathe it in. Allow this fragrance to relax you (more) deeply. Feel the energy of this oil melting away any tension or resistance you may be carrying in your body. Breathe in relaxation; breathe out tension. With your next inhalation, allow your awareness to float to the crown of your head. As you exhale, relax from your crown all the way down through your body into your toes. Feel each breath helping your muscles unwind. Continue like this for a few minutes: breathing in to the top of your head, breathing out all the way down into your toes.

Now, bring your awareness to your belly and feel your baby inside your womb. Breathe peacefulness into your belly and relax with your baby as you breathe out.

Conscious Choice Making

You are the sum total of the choices you make. At a very basic level, the choices you make determine your sensory experience—what you hear, feel, see, taste, and smell. When you are in touch with the inner experiences that result from sensations you intake from the world, you are in touch with the core of your life. Every experience has an impact on your biology. Everything that has happened to you is recorded in your body; with each new experience, your body changes. The more consciously you choose your experiences, the more consciously you create your body.

Pregnancy is not just something that is happening to you; it is a miraculous unfolding that you are co-creating. For nine months, you are your unborn baby's environment, and your baby is affected by each one of your experiences. At the core of your being you already know this, because you have had this experience and felt these sensations as you developed and grew inside your mother's womb. Now that this information is available to your conscious mind, make use of it to create a magical beginning for your child.

Enliven Through Your Attention

- Place your hands on your belly a few times throughout the day and send loving thoughts to your unborn baby.
- Journal each day about your experiences.

• Early in your pregnancy, plant a tree or flowering bush to symbolize the growth of your baby in your womb. After your child is born, you can take care of the plant together.

• Read enchanting stories and heartfelt poetry aloud to your baby and listen to beautiful, relaxing music each day.

• Perform a daily oil massage on yourself before you bathe or shower.

• Diffuse an aroma while listening to music, while soaking in a tub, or while meditating to create the association between the fragrance and the relaxed state of awareness.

CHAPTER 3

Nourishment for Two

From Cosmic intelligence came space;

From space, air;

From air, fire;

From fire, water;

From water, plants;

From plants, food;

And from food the human body,

Heads, arms, legs and heart.

—TAITTIRIYA UPANISHAD

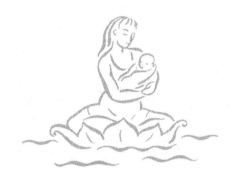

rom your earliest childhood, you are barraged with messages about food. In addition to the basic information transmitted by your parents, you've received thousands of hours of propaganda from television, radio, roadside advertisements, and print media, all attempting to shape your eating habits. Considering the volume of advice you've been exposed to, it's not surprising that you might be confused about what to eat. It is also not unexpected that since so many people have lost touch with their intrinsic body intelligence, we are facing an epidemic of obesity in our society.

Ayurveda suggests that the wisdom of nature is available in every cell of your body, and if you listen to the messages your body is sending, you will naturally eat a healthy and balanced diet. We view the Ayurvedic approach as nature speaking directly to us. Your senses are created to perceive those things in the world that are nourishing to you. Your ability to taste, smell, and see potential food sources provides the natural clues as to what to favor in your diet and what to reduce. Paying attention to flavors, aromas, and colors in your diet will ensure that you are ingesting the foods you need in order to create a healthy body for you and your unborn baby.

Ayurveda holds that nutrition involves more than what you ingest by way of protein, carbohydrates, and fats. Nutrition is the process by which Mother Nature packages energy and information into vegetables, grains, fruits, and nuts that are then metabolized by animals into the energy and information of their bodies. Most fundamentally, food is sunlight condensed into matter.

An ancient Vedic hymn declares, "Food is Brahman," which means "Food is Intelligence." When we consume food derived from the union of natural sunlight, fertile earth, pure water, and clean air, our bodies, emotions, and souls are nourished. We inherently recognize the relationship between food and our hearts and souls, as evidenced by our language, which frequently uses flavors and food as metaphors for feelings and emotions. We use expressions such as "sweet love," "sour grapes," and "acid tones." We describe our true emotions as "gut feelings" and tell our children they are so cute "we could eat them up."

The process of creating a body from food is miraculous. Ayurveda describes the body as DNA wrapped with food. The DNA from you and your partner merges to create your baby, providing the template to weave the energy and information of the environment into your baby's physical body. When you consume a four-course Italian meal, the minestrone soup, spinach salad, pasta, tomato sauce, string beans, garlic bread, and cannoli carry both energy, in the form of calories, and information, in the form of vitamins, minerals, and natural chemicals. You digest, absorb, and metabolize the energy and information of your food into the intelligence of your body.

Simultaneously your unborn baby extracts and metabolizes the nutritional information in your bloodstream into his developing body. Carotene molecules inside a carrot in your soup become woven into the retina of your baby's eyes. Essential fatty acids from the olive oil in your salad dressing make up the cell membranes of your baby's liver. Your baby's body is manufactured from the food you eat. Although it is true throughout one's life, it becomes particularly important during pregnancy to consume a healthy, balanced, delicious diet. Fortunately, with a little attention, this is easy to accomplish. The principles are simple: throughout the day, eat foods that carry the six basic flavors your taste buds are capable of identifying and the seven basic colors your eyes are designed to recognize. By paying attention to the six tastes and seven colors, your diet will be delicious and nutritionally complete.

The Six Tastes of Life

From the standpoint of Ayurveda, all sources of potential nourishment can be categorized according to one or more of six basic flavors. These are *sweet, sour, salty, pungent, bitter,* and *astringent.* The basic strategy, which holds true whether or not you are pregnant, is to have foods representing all six tastes in your diet on a daily basis. This will ensure that you maintain the appropriate balance of carbohydrates, protein, and fat along with abundant levels of essential vitamins and minerals. Variety is the key to a healthy, balanced diet. Let's review each taste in more detail.

SWEET

If you listen to your body, during pregnancy you will naturally be attracted to sweet foods. This does not imply that you will be consuming large quantities of refined sugar. Any food that is nourishing and brings satisfaction has a sweet component. Sweetness is characteristic of bulk-building foods. Sweet foods are abundant sources of energy, but poorer sources of information. The energy component of foods is quantified by measuring calories. Foods that are calorically rich contain carbohydrates, protein, and fat. Each gram of carbohydrate and protein carries about four calories, while each gram of fat contains nine calories.

The sweet category of foods includes milk, cheese, butter, nuts, tofu, breads, pasta, grains, starchy vegetables, sweet fruits, oils, and all animal products. In addition to their mass-building properties, sweet foods are soothing and have a softening effect on tissues. If you look at your grocery cart in the checkout line, you will recognize that foods carrying the sweet taste constitute the largest component of a healthy diet. A healthy balance of foods in this category is essential to supply adequate protein, essential fatty acids, and calories to your developing baby.

SOUR

Sour taste is a feature of organic acids. Citric acid and ascorbic acid, found in citrus fruits, berries, and tomatoes; lactic acid, found in cheese and yogurt; and acetic acid, present in pickles and salad dressings, all carry the sour taste. Sour foods aid in digestion, stimulate the appetite, and help move food through the digestive tract. A healthy diet includes regular doses of the sour taste, primarily through the intake of fruits, berries, and tomatoes. Sweet fruits such as apples, apricots, grapes, plums, and pineapples also carry the sour flavor. Sour-carrying fruits provide essential quantities of vitamin C and flavonoids, which are necessary for healthy cell development and normal immune function.

SALTY

We emerged from the ocean millions of years ago and still carry it in our blood. Salty is the flavor of the ocean and we have an inherent impulse to seek out sources of salt in our diet. In Western society you are much more likely to get too much rather than too little salt in your diet, but your systems could not function without a daily helping of sodium chloride. In addition to table salt, which should be used sparingly, the salty taste is carried in soy sauce, seafood, and seaweed products. In addition to its water-retaining properties, salty foods enhance digestion and are mildly sedating and laxative.

PUNGENT

The pungent flavor is most commonly referred to as "hot" or "spicy." The pungent taste results from essential oils that stimulate the mucous membranes. These oils have been found to be rich in antioxidants, which explains why spices have been used for millennia to preserve food. The pungent flavor stimulates digestion, helps relieve nausea, cleanses the sinuses and respiratory tract, and is mildly laxative. Many foods carry the pungent flavor—including onions, leeks, garlic, scallions, chives, radishes, and chili peppers. Many of these foods have been shown to help reduce serum cholesterol levels, lower blood pressure, and enhance immune function. In addition, many culinary spices such as cloves, cinnamon, cayenne, black pepper, thyme, oregano, rosemary, basil, and nutmeg are mildly to moderately pungent and are flavor-enhancing and health-promoting additions to every diet.

One of the most important pungent spices is gingerroot. This prized medicinal and culinary spice has been used around the world to stimulate digestion and ease nausea. Studies using gingerroot in the treatment of morning sickness have shown it to be moderately effective. Since you will want to avoid any unnecessary medications during pregnancy, drinking ginger tea or chewing on a small piece of gingerroot can be a safe and effective way to relieve the distressing nausea so commonly experienced in the first trimester. Western diets tend to be rather weak when it comes to the spicy taste, but there is abundant evidence to suggest that adding a little pungency to your meals is good for your taste buds and your physiology.

BITTER

Bitter is the flavor of green and yellow vegetables. Their bitter taste is due to the stimulation of specific receptors on the tongue that monitor the levels of certain chemicals in your food. Many of the most important natural health-promoting constituents of vegetables, known as phytonutrients or phytochemicals (*phyto* is Latin for "plant") have a bitter taste. These include natural disease-fighting, immune-enhancing, and growth-promoting substances such as flavonoids, polyphenols, and terpenes.

Bitter foods include broccoli, chard, eggplant, spinach, and zucchini. Leafy greens are considered bitter, as are many common culinary and medicinal herbs, such as dill, fenugreek, sage, and chamomile. The bitter taste can stimulate digestion and has a detoxifying effect on the system.

ASTRINGENT

Astringent foods have a puckering or drying effect on mucous membranes. Western nutrition does not usually consider astringency as a separate taste, but the chemicals responsible for this "puckering" effect have many health-enhancing benefits. Foods with an astringent flavor include tart apples, asparagus, green peppers, cranberries, pomegranates, and spinach. Some of the best astringent foods are beans and legumes. Lentils, chickpeas, soybeans, and split peas are excellent sources of vegetable protein, complex carbohydrates, and fiber. They also provide healthy doses of calcium, magnesium, and folic acid.

At the turn of the twentieth century, vegetable sources of protein from nuts, beans, and peas made up a much higher portion of the American diet. Over the past hundred years we have substantially replaced most of these vegetable sources of protein with animal ones. Along with this shift we've seen a marked rise in the risk of heart disease and various cancers. There is abundant evidence to suggest that reducing your intake of animal protein and increasing high-quality vegetable sources can enhance your current and future health.

The Colors of Food

Phytochemicals are not only responsible for the flavors and smells of your food; they also underlie its color. In his wonderful book *What Color Is Your Diet?*, David Heber, M.D., reminds us that expanding the visual palette of your diet improves its nutritional value. Take on the intention to consume a colorful diet, rich with beautiful vegetables, fruits, beans, and grains, and you will take advantage of the health-promoting intelligence that nature provides. From an evolutionary perspective, one of the reasons you are able to perceive the seven colors of the rainbow is so that you can distinguish a juicy ripe red strawberry from an unripe one or a delicious yellow banana from a green one. The average Western diet with its emphasis on browns and beiges tends to be rather bland from a visual as well as nutritional perspective. Examples of foods of various colors are given below. You'll notice that we naturally eat many red, orange, yellow, and green foods, but it takes more attention to find foods on the blue side of the color spectrum. Enrich your diet with color, and you enrich it with nutrients as well.

Colorful Nutrition

COLOR	EXAMPLES
Red	Strawberries, red bell peppers, pink grapefruit, tomatoes, watermelon, beets, radishes
Orange	Oranges, cantaloupe, carrots, apricots, mango
Yellow	Yellow squash, bananas, onions, peaches, millet
Green	Broccoli, zucchini, spinach, green beans, chard, lima beans
Blue	Blueberries, blue corn
Indigo	Eggplant, blackberries, plums, prunes, black beans
Violet	Grapes, kale, purple potatoes, purple basil

A Balanced Pregnancy Diet

Pregnancy is not a time for radical nutrition. Regardless of your personal dietary choices, you have an obligation to ensure that your food selections are fully nourishing to your unborn baby. The essence of parenting is stretching your boundaries for the benefit of your offspring. If you need to be either more expansive or more selective in your eating practices so your baby-to-be creates a healthy body, view these changes as an opportunity to cultivate flexibility—a trait that will serve you well in child rearing.

There are a few basic principles that apply to nutrition during pregnancy. Be creative in how you follow these principles, but remember that your diet is your unborn baby's diet.

1. EAT NUTRITIOUS FOOD.

In the later months of your pregnancy, you may find that your capacity for food diminishes due to pressure on digestive organs from your growing womb. Cultivate the habit early so that you don't waste calories on nutritionally empty food. Rather than indulging on chips and cookies, favor fruits, yogurt, and whole-grain cereals. This does not mean that you cannot enjoy a daily delicious treat; simply be conscious of the nutritional value of everything you allow into your body.

2. LISTEN TO YOUR APPETITE.

During most of the nineteenth century and the first half of the twentieth, pregnant women were told to restrict their food intake and limit their weight gain. As a result, problems associated with low-birth-weight babies were common, including increased susceptibility to infection and delayed neurological development. The injunction to limit weight gain derived from the recognition that small babies are easier to deliver than large ones.

We now know that a well-balanced nutritional program naturally leads to bigger, healthier babies. In general, a weight gain of 25 to 35 pounds leads to the healthiest newborns. These extra pounds are composed of the following:

Baby: 7½ pounds
Uterus: 2½-pound weight gain
Placenta: 1 pound
Amniotic fluid: 2 pounds
Mother's breasts: 3-pound weight gain
Mother's blood: 4-pound increase
Mother's fat: 5+ pound increase
Total weight gain: 25+ pounds

Listening to your appetite is the best way to ensure that you add weight at the right rate, which is a few pounds during the first trimester and about a pound per week for the remainder of the pregnancy. Listening to your appetite means eating when you are hungry and stopping when you are comfortably satisfied. A useful way to consider your appetite is by envisioning a satiety gauge, where 0 is completely empty and 10 is stuffed. The general rule is to eat when you are at level 3 and stop when you are at level 7. Level 3 means you are very hungry and thinking about food, but not having hunger pangs. Level 7 means you are comfortably full, but still have about a third of your stomach empty. Avoiding the impulse to eat until you are stuffed maximizes your digestive power and ensures you are getting the appropriate caloric intake.

3. CONSUME ADEQUATE AMOUNTS OF HIGH-QUALITY PROTEIN.

Protein-rich foods supply the essential amino acids that are necessary for healthy fetal development. Proteins are indispensable components of cells, enzymes, and many hormones. The protein you ingest is broken down in your stomach and the early part of your small intestines. The resultant amino acids are absorbed farther down the digestive tract and assembled into the essential structures of your body and the body of your unborn baby.

The recommended intake of protein for a pregnant woman is approximately .5 grams per pound of body weight. If you weigh 120 pounds, you should be eating about 60 grams of protein per day ($0.5 \times 120 = 60$). Examples of the protein content of different foods are listed below.

Protein Contents

FOOD	QUANTITY	GRAMS OF PROTEIN
Milk	1 cup	9
Cottage cheese	2 ounces	9
Egg	1 whole	6
Beans or peas	½ cup dried, cooked	8
Roasted nuts	¼ cup	6–7
Peanut butter	1 tbsp	4
Vegetables	½ cup	1–3
Fruits	½ cup	1–2
Pasta or rice	½ cup, cooked	2
Bread, wheat	1 slice	2–3
Fish, fowl, meat	3 ounces, cooked	15–25

Your body is unable to synthesize eight essential amino acids in adequate amounts and, therefore, you must ingest them from outside food sources. All eight of these amino acids are present in dairy and animal products, but one or more are usually deficient in vegetable protein sources. This does not mean that you cannot get sufficient high-quality protein on a pure vegan diet, but it does mean that you must be extremely careful to combine abundant amounts of beans, nuts, whole grains, fruits, and vegetables. If you are vegetarian, it is much easier and safer to follow a lacto-ovo diet during pregnancy, consuming regular doses of dairy products and eggs. In the interest of your

environment, your unborn baby, and yourself, consume
only organic milk, cheese, and yogurt, and eggs from
free-ranging, hormone-free chickens.

4. CONSUME FOODS THAT CONTAIN BOTH OMEGA-3 AND OMEGA-6 FATTY ACIDS.

Essential fatty acids are required for the normal
development of the fetal nervous system and immune
system. The fetus extracts the required fats from the
circulation of Mother, who must consume them in her
diet. There are two main categories of essential fats,
commonly known as omega-3 and omega-6 fatty acids.
Most Western diets are high in omega-6 but relatively
deficient in omega-3 fatty acids. Omega-6 fatty acids
are abundant in most seed- and nut-derived oils, such
as almond, corn, safflower, sesame, sunflower, and
walnut. Seed oils contain relatively low levels of
omega-3 fatty acids with the exception of flaxseed,
canola, and soybean. Most green vegetables are rich in
omega-3 fatty acids, but since there is so little fat in
vegetables, the total dose of omega-3 fatty acids from
vegetables is limited.

Fish oils contain abundant quantities of omega-3
fatty acids, but there is increasing concern that
predatory fish (shark, swordfish, king mackerel, and
tilefish) along with freshwater fish contain potentially
hazardous levels of the toxin methylmercury. The Food
and Drug Administration has advised pregnant women

to avoid eating these fish and to limit their intake of other seafood to 12 ounces per week. Tuna is in the gray zone because larger tuna that are sold for steaks have higher concentrations of mercury, whereas the smaller tuna most often used for canned fish have lower levels. Mercury released from industrial sites enters our water supply through the air and soil and becomes concentrated in fish. It has been shown that the consumption of mercury-containing fish by pregnant women can lead to toxic levels, which may impair neurological development in their unborn babies.

The bottom line is to put attention on adding omega-3 food sources to your diet. Cook with canola or soybean oil, add roasted flaxseeds to your salads and sautéed vegetables, and eat a few walnuts every day. If you eat fish, do not overdo it and avoid those that are known to carry a higher risk for mercury contamination.

5. TAKE A HIGH-QUALITY PRENATAL VITAMIN SUPPLEMENT THROUGHOUT YOUR PREGNANCY. Even with the best intentions to eat a balanced diet, you do not want to risk a nutritional deficiency while you are pregnant. Many of your essential nutrient needs rise during pregnancy, including increased requirements for calcium, magnesium, phosphorus, iron, and vitamin D. Your need for antioxidant vitamins (A, C, E) rises by 10 to 20 percent. With the increased metabolic activity of

pregnancy comes a slightly increased requirement for the B vitamins. One of the B vitamins, folic acid, has been identified as a critical nutrient, which if deficient can lead to developmental defects in the brain and spinal cord. Supplementation with folic acid is considered prudent; most prenatal daily vitamins contain 800 mcg of it.

All essential vitamins and minerals are necessary for a healthy baby, but it is possible to overdose. Too much vitamin A has been associated with a variety of birth defects, so current recommendations are to consume less than 10,000 international units (IUs) per day. Between a balanced diet and a good standard prenatal vitamin, you will easily ensure that both you and your baby are well nourished. Discuss with your health care advisor his or her vitamin recommendations, but don't substitute good vitamins for good food.

Eating with Awareness

From a mind-body perspective, nutrition is not limited to just the food we consume. The environment in which we dine, our emotional state, and the conversations we engage in during the meal are as essential to optimal nutrition as the food we are eating. How we eat is as important as what we eat. Try the exercise on page 90 to have a clear experience of how it feels to eat mindfully.

Vitamin and Mineral Intake During Pregnancy

NUTRIENT	RECOMMENDED DAILY ALLOWANCE (RDA)	STANDARD PRENATAL VITAMIN SUPPLEMENT
Vitamin A	4000 IU	2500–5000 IU
Vitamin D	400 IU	400 IU
Vitamin E	24 IU	30 IU
Vitamin C	60 mg	60–120 mg
Vitamin B_1 (*Thiamin*)	1.1 mg	1.6–3 mg
Vitamin B_2 (*Riboflavin*)	1.3 mg	1.8–3.4 mg
Niacinamide	15 mg	17–20 mg
Vitamin B_6 (*Pyridoxine*)	1.6 mg	4 mg
Folate	400 mcg	800 mcg
Vitamin B_{12}	2 mcg	12 mcg
Calcium	1200 mg	200–250 mg
Magnesium	280 mg	100 mg
Iron	15 mg	28–90 mg
Zinc	12 mg	25 mg
Iodine	150 mcg	150–200 mcg
Copper	2 mg	2–3 mg

IU = international units • mg = milligrams • mcg = micrograms

Exercise

This is a fun exercise to do with a partner or friend. Select three different types of food to use for this exercise. For example, you might select an orange slice, a few raisins, and some sunflower seeds. Group your choices into three separate piles.

Close your eyes and sit quietly for a few minutes. Feel yourself breathing in and out and allow your body to relax. Notice the space inside your body and keep breathing into your inner space until you feel settled. Now open your eyes and select a piece of food. Look at it closely and notice its color and texture. What does it feel like as you hold it between your fingers? Notice its aroma. Slowly close your eyes and put this piece of food into your mouth. Feel the sensations as it enters your body. Notice the flavor and texture as you begin to chew. Experience the sensations of your tongue moving the food inside your mouth. Do you like or dislike the taste? Is this flavor triggering any memories? Wait until the bite is completely liquefied before you swallow it. Can you feel it moving down your esophagus into your stomach? How full is your stomach?

Once you are finished with your first bite, sit quietly for a few moments and reflect on what you noticed. You may, for example, discover that flavors and textures are more vibrant. Reflect on what it feels like to be present to each aspect of eating. When you feel ready, try another type of food. Repeat the same process. Notice all the sensations that this new food brings to your awareness. Savor each bite. After you have swallowed, sit quietly once again. When you are ready, try the last type of food. Notice the differences and similarities in tastes, sensations, aromas, and memories evoked by each piece of food. When you feel ready, open your eyes and share your experience with your partner.

Practice eating with awareness. Most of us do not take the time to just sit and eat. We are too busy eating and doing, eating and talking, eating and working, even eating and driving. We forget that eating is a delightful experience in itself, worthy of our full attention. When you eat with awareness, you will notice how each bite nourishes your body, mind, and soul. Choose one meal this week to eat in silence, noticing the flavors, sensations, and aromas that nurture you.

Body Intelligence Techniques for Pregnancy

Here are some suggestions to help expand your enjoyment at each meal.

- Eat your meals in a peaceful and settled environment. Avoid eating when you are upset.
- Eliminate alcohol, nicotine, and nonprescription drugs from your life.
- Make an effort to eliminate or cut back on caffeine, remembering that chocolate and soft drinks often contain caffeine.

• Honor your appetite. You may get hungry many times per day, particularly later in your pregnancy. Eat when you feel hungry and stop when you are satiated.

• Don't overeat; leave about a third of your stomach empty to aid digestion.

• Eat at a comfortable pace; stay conscious of the process.

• Eat freshly prepared foods. Lightly cooked foods are preferable to raw or overcooked foods.

• Favor fruits, vegetables, and grains.

• Favor low-fat dairy, almonds, and honey.

• Reduce ice-cold foods and beverages.

• Drink plenty of pure, room-temperature water each day.

• Sit quietly for a few minutes after finishing your meal.

• Honor any cravings you may have, but indulge in them with awareness.

• Include all six tastes at every meal.

• Comply with any supplementary vitamins recommended by your health provider.

With each bite of food, you ingest a universe of experiences. Many things conspired to create the carrots on your plate—the rain, sunshine, and clouds, the plants and animals in the ecosystem of the carrot farm, the farmer and his relationships, the soil, insects, worms, and birds, the production plant, the truck drivers, the food market, and the produce manager. The more you consider how much is involved in the creation of your foods, the more you must marvel at the web of life and how you and your baby are inextricably woven into it. Be mindful as you choose the food you eat, for you are not only choosing for yourself, you are choosing for your unborn baby as well.

Enliven Through Your Attention

• Place your hands on your belly a few times throughout the day and send loving thoughts to your unborn baby.

• Journal each day about your experiences.

• Early in your pregnancy, plant a tree or flowering bush to symbolize the growth of your baby in the womb. After your child is born, you can take care of the plant together.

• Read enchanting stories and heartfelt poetry aloud to your baby and listen to beautiful, relaxing music each day.

• Perform a daily oil massage on yourself before you bathe or shower.

• Diffuse an aroma while listening to music, while soaking in a tub, or while meditating to create the association between the fragrance and the relaxed state of awareness.

• Ensure that you have all six tastes available during your meals throughout the day.

• Choose to eat meals that are rich in color, aroma, and texture.

• Be mindful as you eat your meals. Eat at least one meal each week in silence with your full awareness.

CHAPTER 4

Maintaining Your Balance

There is nothing as ancient as infancy.

Unchanging ancientness is born into homes

Again and again in the form of a baby;

Yet, the freshness, beauty, innocence and sweetness

It had at the beginning of history

Is the same today.

—RABINDANATH TAGORE

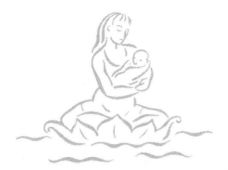

*Y*our unborn baby has a direct connection to your thoughts and emotions. As a result of this intimate communication link, the expectant family assumes a new responsibility. For the benefit of both your unborn baby and your family, it is essential that you cultivate the ability to maintain your balance while facing the inevitable daily stresses of life. Learning to stay centered during the ups and downs will serve you well throughout your pregnancy and throughout your life.

We have learned a lot about stress over the past seventy

years. Whenever you feel physically or emotionally threatened, your body and mind shift into a protective mode. Your heart beats faster and harder. You breathe more rapidly. Your adrenal glands squirt out stress hormones including adrenaline and cortisol, and your blood sugar rises. Your body perspires and your blood clots a little easier. These physiological changes prepare you to deal aggressively with the stress, either by fighting or running away. This reaction has become known as the fight-or-flight response. If the source of your stress is a wild tiger trying to eat you for lunch, the impulse to pick up a stick or run up a tree is adaptive and potentially life saving. If the source of your stress is a traffic jam during rush hour or a delayed airplane flight, activating the fight-or-flight response does you little good.

Eliciting the stress response repeatedly over time eventually predisposes you to illness ranging from chronic fatigue to heart disease.

Studies have shown that when you inject the stress hormones adrenaline and noradrenaline into a calm animal, it reacts as if it were facing a stressful threat. The animal's heart races, its blood pressure rises, and it appears to be agitated. When a pregnant mother is anxious, stressed, or in a fearful state, the stress hormones released into her bloodstream cross through the placenta to the baby. The unborn baby responds to her mother's stress in a similar way.

A study by an obstetrician from Austria, Dr. Emil Reinold, explored how quickly a mother's anxiety elicits a response in the unborn baby. Reinold instructed a group of pregnant women that he was going to check their baby with an ultrasound machine. After asking them to lie down and relax, and letting them know he was waiting for the baby to become calm, he told the mothers (knowing his statement would elicit anxiety) that the baby wasn't moving. In every case, within seconds after the mothers received this information, their babies began kicking strongly.

In the early 1980s after an earthquake in Italy, pregnant women were studied by ultrasound. Each mother was anxious and frightened as a result of the earthquake, and their unborn babies had become unusually active in response to their mothers' stress. Most of these babies remained agitated for several hours after the incident, and then many became inactive for up to three days before settling back into their normal rate of activity. Under intense maternal stress, the fetus activates its own fight-or-flight response, at times becoming exhausted.

In our Magical Beginnings courses taught at the Chopra Center, we ask pregnant mothers attending our childbirth classes to observe their stresses for a week, noticing if their babies show any response. Mothers consistently report that when they feel stressed, their babies often react by kicking. They repeatedly notice that loud noises such as dogs barking, sirens sounding, horns honking, and people yelling cause their babies to react. The unborn baby is a conscious, sentient being with thoughts, feelings, and memories of her own. She can experience pleasure, pain, fear, stress, and serenity, in response to his mother's experiences and reactions.

Hundreds of studies have confirmed that chemicals released by the pregnant mother's body are transported into the womb and affect the unborn baby. Maternal stress influences uterine blood flow. Stress activates the unborn child's endocrine system and influences fetal brain development. Children born to mothers who had intensely stressful pregnancies are more likely to have behavioral problems later in life. These studies do not suggest that every time you get upset about something, you are harming your unborn baby. Rather, we hope that they will motivate you to deal with your daily challenges with as balanced a state of mind as possible.

A neonatologist friend of ours, Dr. Jamison Jones, tells the story of two premature infants under his care. Born two months early, they were in the neonatal intensive care unit at the same time. One was the baby of a woman who was a heroin addict. The other was born to a high-powered executive who worked up until the day she went into premature labor. Although these two babies came from mothers of vastly different socioeconomic backgrounds, they demonstrated similar problems in the hospital. Each had accelerated heart rates and difficulty breathing and appeared highly agitated. Although they were incubated in mothers from very different worlds, they had one thing in common: both mothers were under a tremendous amount of stress during the pregnancy.

Your unborn baby cannot control your choices or reactions to the world and therefore cannot control the sensations she experiences. If you are experiencing stress, your baby experiences it along with you. Stresses can be emotional or physical. In a fascinating study published by Dr. Michael Lieberman, unborn babies' responses to their mothers' smoking were monitored. He found that the babies became agitated within a few seconds after their mothers inhaled. The babies' heart rates, kicking movements, and breathing motions all increased. Of even greater significance was the observation that when these mothers simply thought of having a cigarette, the babies had similar agitated responses.

We cannot ensure that our lives are stress free, but we can learn to reduce our reactivity to life challenges. Just as our body/minds are wired to respond to threats in an aggressive manner, we have the capacity to respond with restful awareness to circumstances throughout the day. Learning to be mindful of the situations that trigger your stressful reactions is an important first step in reducing them.

Managing Stress

Exercise

Over the course of a week notice the situations, circumstances, people, and events that trigger your feelings of stress. Each time you observe yourself reacting, shift into a witnessing mode. Identify where you feel the sensation of stress inside your body and notice if your baby kicks or has another response to your stress. Keep your journal handy so you can record your observations.

After a week's worth of journaling, find a quiet place and, with your journal, markers, and pen, draw a stick figure portrait of yourself on the center of a page of paper. Draw a picture of your baby growing inside your womb. While rereading your observations of the situations and circumstances that catalyzed your upsets, notice where in your body you feel your stress. Use your markers to identify these places on your stick figure, choosing a different color for each stressful situation. Next to each location where you marked your stressful feelings, write a few words to describe them. To reinforce the connection between your feelings and those of your unborn baby, draw lines from the stressful sites in your body to your pregnant belly.

As you look at your portrait, think about your baby, your body, and the ways you can reduce your stress. Consider how you can best nourish and take care of yourself and your baby each day. Take a few moments to journal your thoughts.

Below we offer some suggestions to reduce the harmful effects of stress on you and your baby.

- When you feel the sensation of stress, take in a few long, slow breaths. Feel yourself bringing oxygen into your body and imagine it infusing your baby.
- Massage your belly when you notice that you are feeling stressed. As you rub your belly, let your baby know that both of you are okay.
- Take time out of each day to relax quietly.
- Take walks in nature.

- Soak in a warm aroma bath.
- Listen to music that makes you feel happy.
- Snuggle up with your partner or a close friend.
- Get some form of exercise daily.
- Treat yourself to a massage.
- Practice meditation.

Finding Silence/Releasing Stress

What is the value of meditation for parents-to-be? There are benefits on many levels. From a basic physiological perspective, meditation is the perfect antidote to stress. During a stressful encounter your heart rate and blood pressure rise, your breathing becomes rapid and shallow, and your adrenal glands pump out stress hormones. During meditation, your heart rate slows, your blood pressure normalizes, your breathing quiets, and your stress hormone levels fall. Meditation enhances both mental and physical health.

I have never encountered another temple as blissful as my own body.

—SARAHA

When a mother takes the time to quiet her mind and center herself, the calming physiological changes that are invoked through meditation are also communicated to the baby. Stress hormone levels fall, oxygenation improves, and the unborn baby gains the psychological and physiological benefits of restful awareness.

Outside of the actual practice time, meditation helps you become less reactive to stressful encounters. Many studies have shown that people who meditate regularly are more adaptable both mentally and physically to life's challenges. Meditators have less anxiety and depression. They show lower rates of high blood pressure and are less likely to use prescription or nonprescription drugs to regulate their moods. Taking the opportunity to connect with a deeper aspect of your being enables you to be more centered, less reactive, more responsive, less anxious, more creative, and less habitual in all aspects of your life. As a result of this expanded state of awareness, you are able to use your energy more efficiently and enjoy your life and your family more.

Meditation will help you quiet your inner dialogue so that you can be fully present to your experiences in each moment. This will allow you to be more fully open to yourself transforming as a mother, while bringing mindfulness to your body as you grow and then give birth to your baby. Meditation is the most important tool to expand awareness. It provides you with the opportunity to turn your attention inward. Normally your awareness is directed outward through your senses to the sounds, sensations, sights, tastes, and smells of the world around you. Meditation is the process of disengaging your senses so you can experience the expanded silence within you. This domain of awareness is the source of your thoughts and feelings. Although it is beyond mental activity, it gives rise to all creativity, insight, and understanding. Accessing this field of awareness on a daily basis through meditation encourages your identity to become more expansive, even in the midst of daily life.

In each of our lives we experience a constant influx of change. We can see this in our day-to-day lives, as people come and go, as our feelings, thoughts, and perceptions shift, as we take deeper or shallower breaths, as our body image alters over time, and as each of the seasons changes—all of these aspects of our lives are continually transforming. The challenge is learning to refine our awareness so we can be with each of these experiences fully.

There are many effective techniques of meditation. The essence of meditation is shifting your awareness from the objects of experience to the experiencer. In daily life, your attention constantly moves from one sensory experience to another. You listen to the radio, sip your coffee, read the morning newspaper, feel the accelerator pedal under your foot, hear the conversations over your phone, and smell the strawberries at the market.

My inside,
listen to me,
The greatest
spirit,
The Teacher,
is near,
Wake up,
wake up!
Run to his feet,
He is standing
close to your
head
Right now.
You have slept
for millions
and millions
of years.
Why not wake up
this morning?

—KABIR

Your awareness is continually being seduced outward. During meditation you relinquish your attachment to the experiences of your senses and become intimate with the one who is having the experiences. You shift your reference point from the objects of experience to the alert witness of the experience. Your identity shifts from ego to spirit, from constricted awareness to expanded awareness.

Mantra Meditation

Try this simple meditation technique that uses your breath and a breathing mantra to quiet mental activity and bring you to a state of restful awareness.

Find a quiet place where you will not be disturbed. Turn off the ringer on your phone and let your family know that you would appreciate twenty minutes of privacy. Find a comfortable place to sit with your back supported, but do not support your head. Take a few deep breaths and allow the tension to be released from your body. Close your eyes and simply become aware of the activity of your mind. Notice how your thoughts come and go without any effort on your part. It is the nature of the mind to generate thought forms spontaneously.

Bring your attention to your breathing. Observe the inflow and outflow of your breath without attempting to consciously influence the rate or depth of your breathing. Maintain an attitude of innocence, neither resisting nor anticipating any particular experience. Silently begin repeating the mantra "so-hum" with your breathing. Think the word "so" on your inhalations and "hum" on your exhalations. Silent mental repetition does not involve a clear pronunciation of these sounds. They are faint impulses repeated effortlessly.

At times your attention will drift away from the mantra and become absorbed in a thought. You may at times become aware of sounds in your environment. A sensation in your body may occasionally take your attention from the gentle repetition of the mantra. Whenever you become aware that your attention has drifted away from "so-hum" to another thought, sound, or sensation, gently return your attention to the mantra.

What lies before us and what lies behind us is but a small matter compared to what lies within us.

—RALPH WALDO EMERSON

Continue this procedure for about twenty minutes. When the time is up, allow your awareness to float freely. Wait a couple of minutes before opening your eyes and resuming your activities.

Understanding Your Experiences in Meditation

All experiences during meditation fall into one of four categories: (1) silently repeating the mantra, (2) having thoughts,

(3) falling asleep, or (4) going into the gap between thoughts. Each of these is a sign that you are practicing meditation correctly. Let's review each in more detail.

THE MANTRA

A mantra is a sound with a pleasant vibration that does not engage your intellect. It is a word without meaning, which therefore does not keep your awareness trapped on the level of analysis or understanding. Because the mantra does not trigger the usual associations that normal words do, it acts as a vehicle to experience thought forms at subtler levels of development.

When you place your awareness on the mantra, you may notice that it changes—in rhythm, rate, or clarity. A change in your perception of the mantra suggests that you are experiencing less localized expressions of it; do not resist changes in the mantra. Whenever you recognize that you are no longer repeating the mantra, gently return your awareness to it.

THOUGHTS

When people first start meditating, they often complain that they are having too many thoughts. Although it may not feel very comfortable when your mind is active, being aware of the activity of your mind is an important step. Before beginning meditation, most people never have the thought "I am having too many thoughts." The technology of meditation begins the process of witnessing mental activity. This shift from being caught in your thoughts to becoming the alert witness of thoughts is the shift from ego to spirit.

When you are engrossed in a thought sequence, there is nothing you can do. At some point, however, the thought "I am not thinking the mantra" will arise. When you have this thought, gently shift your attention back to "so-hum."

FALLING ASLEEP

You may fall asleep in your meditation. If you are fatigued and allow yourself the opportunity to relax, your body may take advantage of the opportunity to take a nap. Don't fight the impulse to fall asleep. Allow your body to take the rest it needs. When you awaken, spend at least five minutes thinking the mantra or focusing on your breath so your mind will be clear when you resume your activity.

THE GAP

Finally, you may experience your mind becoming quiet while you maintain full awareness. We describe this experience as slipping into the "gap" between thoughts. Awareness is maintained but there are no objects of awareness. This is the domain of pure consciousness . . . of spirit. Your awareness has gone beyond your environment, beyond your body, and beyond your mind. In this state of pure awareness, you glimpse the reality that your essential nature is not localized in time and space.

Meditation opens your channels of awareness, allowing you entry into a place of peaceful stillness that exists within you. This stillness is your source of happiness, peace, and creativity. As your mind quiets, your body relaxes deeply. Your baby will feel the quietness and relaxation you are generating in your body in her own body.

Raising a child from conception to adulthood will inevitably bring challenges. How you deal with these challenges reflects the quality of your life and shapes the lives of your children. You are not expected to be perfect in the sense that you never feel overwhelmed, frustrated, or irritated, but having a conscious pregnancy and living a conscious life means dedicating yourself to growing in wisdom, peace, harmony, and love. It means making a commitment to learn from your experiences in ways that raise the level of well-being for you and your family. Conscious parenting is a balancing act. As you take on the responsibility of ensuring the safety and nourishment of your children, it is also important to be aware that your children are spiritual beings with their own bodies, minds, souls, and destinies.

The Yoga of Pregnancy

Yoga is a powerful form of exercise that encourages flexibility in the body as well as the mind. If you haven't already experienced yoga, now is the time to do so. Consider it a gift that you give to yourself and to your unborn baby during your pregnancy.

Your yoga practice will reduce your daily stress, thereby

sweetening your inner environment for your baby. As you stretch into poses, you will learn to relax naturally and begin to trust the innate wisdom of your body. Yoga awakens mind/body harmony, making it easier for you to make choices that are good for you both physically and emotionally. Yoga poses can also help relieve many discomforts of pregnancy as they release tension in your body. As you twist and stretch, you will learn to surrender into places that feel tight or out of balance. Your awareness shifts from being in your active mind to being in a deep, quiet place within you.

You will discover that your breath is one of your greatest allies on the journey inward. Yoga helps you listen to your body, your needs, and the needs of your unborn baby. You will find yourself feeling more intuitive and balanced in all aspects of your life, which will help you throughout labor and birth. These yoga poses will enhance your joint flexibility while toning your muscles during pregnancy.

Butterfly Pose

Sit at the edge of a blanket with the heels and soles of your feet together. Pull your feet in toward your body so that they are comfortably close. Rest your hands on your toes or on top of your feet. Close your eyes and lengthen through your spine.

Allow your buttocks to sink down into your blanket. Feel yourself lengthening upward and releasing downward at the same time.

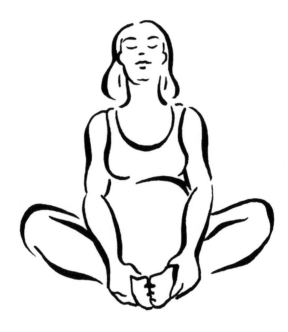

Notice how your thighs begin to soften out to the sides.

Take a few slow, deep breaths, then place your hands on the floor or on a block right in front of your feet. Let your head and neck hang forward, softening your elbows as much as you can and allowing your shoulders to release downward. Take a few slow breaths into your belly, then slide your hands farther forward along the floor until you get to your place of stretch. Let your body sink forward into this stretch and feel your thighs releasing out to the sides even more. Allow the bottom of your spine to soften down toward the earth. Remain in this pose for five to ten slow, relaxed breaths.

To come out of this pose, slowly walk your hands back toward your body and then lengthen your torso, neck, and head until you are back in an upright position.

BENEFITS OF THE BUTTERFLY POSE

Your pelvis consists of four plates of bone joined together by muscle and ligaments. These make up your pelvic girdle. Your baby will be passing through the ring of your pelvic girdle during birth. Throughout pregnancy your body releases hormones that help to soften these ligaments in preparation for birth. The increasing flexibility of your pelvis enables it to shift and widen, making it easier for your baby to maneuver her way through your body as she journeys into the world.

Cat and Cow Pose

Get onto your hands and knees. Your knees should be comfortably apart, with your hands resting beneath your shoulders with palms down and fingers spread wide. Let your neck and head hang forward, while tucking your toes under. Begin to round your buttocks under so that you feel a stretch in your

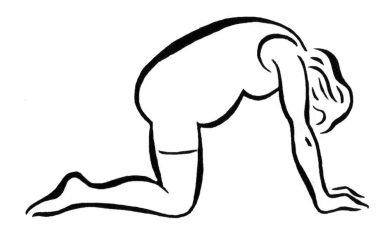

lower back. Press your palms gently into the floor and, starting from your tailbone, begin to round your spine one vertebra at a time up toward the ceiling, and bring your chin in toward your chest. Remain in this rounded position while breathing deeply. Slowly release your body back to center, aligning your head with your spine.

Now, soften your belly, allowing it to sink toward the floor. Simultaneously, begin to tip your buttocks up toward the ceiling, so you create a small arch in your lower back. Lift your head and neck gently upward as though you were peering at someone in front of you. Imagine sending your breath down your spine into your lower back.

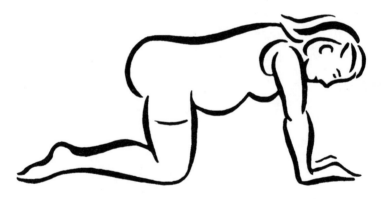

Continue to move back and forth through both parts of this pose—rounding and arching. Notice where you feel tight and where you feel open. Breathe into these places.

BENEFITS OF THE CAT AND COW POSE
This pose increases spinal flexibility and hip mobility. Performing this posture when you are experiencing low back

pain will help stretch the tight muscles that are contributing to your discomfort. Cat and Cow can also be performed during and between labor contractions. It has been suggested that this pose may help rotate babies that are posterior.

Squat Pose

From the hands and knees position in the Cat and Cow Pose, begin to walk your hands back toward your knees. Lift your knees up off the floor. Sink back into your feet and allow your heels to release down toward the floor. If your heels do not rest comfortably, place a folded blanket underneath them. Allow your buttocks to soften and lengthen your tailbone toward your heels.

If you're not comfortable squatting without support, place a rolled blanket between your legs and sit on the blanket in

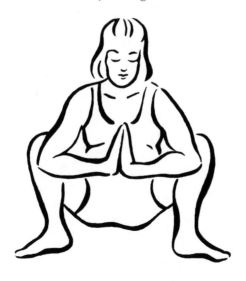

a squatting position. Now clasp your palms and fingers together in front of your heart. Place your elbows between your knees and use your elbows to spread your knees apart. Let your neck and head hang forward comfortably and soften your pelvic floor.

As you take your next inhalation, visualize bringing oxygen and nourishment to you and your baby. As you exhale, allow your pelvic floor to soften. Inhale nourishment and as you exhale release any tightness or tension. Continue for five to ten full, deep breaths.

To come out of this pose, release your clasped hands and elbows, placing one hand and then the other by your buttocks. If you used a rolled blanket, pull it out from under you and sit comfortably on the floor.

SQUATTING FROM A STANDING POSITION
Stand with your feet comfortably apart, placing your hands on your thighs for support. Bend your knees and slowly lower your buttocks down toward the floor. Now clasp your palms and fingers together in front of your heart. Place your elbows between your knees and use your elbows to spread your knees apart. If your heels do not rest comfortably on the floor, place a folded blanket or mat underneath them to support you.

BENEFITS OF THE SQUAT POSE
Women throughout the world assume the squatting pose to give birth. This position widens the pelvis and works with gravity to move the baby through the birth canal. Practiced

during pregnancy, the squat pose relaxes pelvic musculature. Whether or not you decide to give birth in this position, this posture can help ease labor and reduce the chances for tearing of perineal tissue.

Pelvic Tilts

Lie back on your blanket with your feet on the floor and your knees pointing toward the ceiling. Lengthen your neck and allow your shoulders to soften. Allow your arms to rest at your sides. Bring your knees into alignment with your hips. Press weight into your heels and lift your buttocks off the floor as high as you can, pressing your pubic bone toward the ceiling.

Stretch your knees out over your toes as your buttocks continue to lift. Soften your head, neck, shoulders, and arms and take a few long, slow breaths.

Now from your upper back begin to lower your spine, releasing one vertebra at a time until your buttocks are rest-

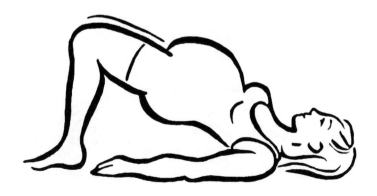

ing comfortably on the floor. Repeat this motion four or five times.

BENEFITS OF PELVIC TILTS

This is another useful posture to improve spinal flexibility and relieve congestion in the lower back muscles. It also helps to improve circulation in the pelvic area and massages your internal organs.

Pigeon Pose

Begin on your hands and knees. Crawl your right knee forward between your hands and slide your right heel toward your left hip. Extend your left leg back behind you, keeping the top of your foot and knee facing the floor. While still supported by your hands, begin to allow your hips and pelvis to release downward. Slowly lower down onto your forearms.

If you find you need more room for your belly and baby, slide your right forearm toward the inside of your right knee. Place a rolled blanket under your arms, hips, or buttocks if you'd like more support. Allow your head and neck to hang

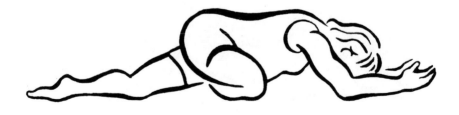

forward to increase the stretch. Turn your elbows out to the sides and allow your head to rest on top of your hands. Breathe and release into the stretch for five to ten breaths.

Repeat the pose on the other side.

BENEFITS OF THE PIGEON POSE
This pose helps stretch and lengthen the muscles around your hips and groin.

Child's Pose

Starting on your hands and knees, move your folded blanket in front of you. Spread your knees apart to create room for your baby. Your feet should be facing inward with the toes of both feet close to each other. Press your buttocks back into your heels and allow your lower spine to lengthen. Bend your elbows and come down onto your forearms. If you are comfortable, stretch your arms farther forward over your blanket. Rest your forehead on the edge of your blanket making sure that you can breathe easily. Soften your neck, shoulders, torso, belly, lower back, and buttocks for five to ten breaths.

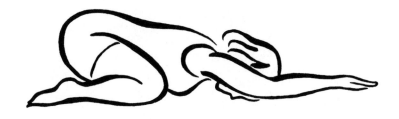

Bring your awareness to your baby and imagine your breath flowing around her.

To come out of the Child's Pose, place your palms by your shoulders, then press into your palms and lift your head and torso. Finally, come all the way back to an upright position.

BENEFITS OF THE CHILD'S POSE

This is a resting pose that helps to release tension in your back muscles and hips, while allowing your belly muscles to soften and relax. It helps to enhance the flexibility of your pelvic joints as it widens the space through your pelvis.

Simple Twist

Sit on the edge of a folded blanket with your legs crossed in front of you. Place your right hand behind you on your blanket with the base of your palm by your buttocks. Press into your palm and lengthen your spine. Reach your left hand across your body and rest it on your right knee. Inhale deeply. As you release your breath, begin twisting your torso to the right beginning with your waist. Continue twisting through your chest, shoulder, neck, and chin. Taking another deep breath, see if you can twist a little farther.

To come out of the pose, soften your back arm and gently allow your torso to return to center. Then repeat the procedure twisting to the left side.

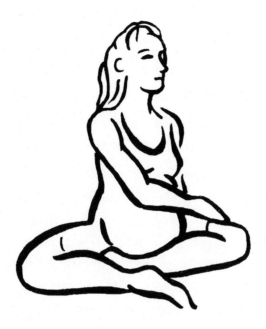

BENEFITS OF THE SIMPLE TWIST

During this pose your internal abdominal organs are massaged while your spinal muscles gently stretch. People often report a sense of enhanced vitality after performing this pose in both directions.

Rotated Stomach Pose

Lie down on the floor on your back. Bend your knees and bring them in toward your chest, resting your arms at your sides with your palms facing up. Roll your hips and bent legs all the way over to the left and allow your legs to rest on the floor, with your thighs resting at a comfortable angle in relationship to your belly.

Rest your left hand on your right leg to give it some support. If your knees do not touch or if you want more support for your legs, place a folded blanket or a pillow in between your thighs. Turn your neck and head away from your knees, and allow your right shoulder to soften toward the floor. If your right arm is uncomfortable, bend the right elbow and place your right hand on your ribs to support them or place a blanket under your ribs and arm for more support.

Take a few slow breaths into your belly and allow your right shoulder to soften toward the floor. Remain in this pose for five to ten breaths, and then roll your legs back to center so that you are again lying on your back. Place your arms around your knees and rock your hips slowly from side to side. Then repeat the process by rolling your body to the right side.

BENEFITS OF THE ROTATED STOMACH POSE
This is a soothing pose for your whole body. It aids digestion and elimination by gently massaging your internal organs. It also helps you stretch and relieve discomfort in your lower and mid-back muscles, and may help relieve discomfort from sciatica.

Kegel Exercises (Pelvic Floor Toners)

Your pelvic floor muscles provide support for your pelvic and abdominal organs. During pregnancy the pelvic floor muscles support your expanding uterus and baby. You can consciously learn to strengthen these muscles by contracting and releasing them throughout the day.

For this exercise we will do the pelvic floor exercises sitting crossed-legged but you can do Kegel exercises anywhere and in any position.

ELEVATOR KEGEL

Sitting with your legs crossed, close your eyes and bring your awareness to your pelvic floor—the space surrounding your urethra, vagina, and anus. Contract the muscles around your anus and then around your vagina and urethra. Continue to contract these muscles inward and upward toward your belly. Imagine moving your energy from your pelvic floor to your abdomen as if traveling up an elevator. Hold for a few breaths, then slowly release the muscles as though you were traveling back down the elevator to the first floor.

Now focus on how your muscles feel back at the pelvic floor and see if you can soften and release them even more. Continue to release these muscles, feeling them relax and open.

THE WAVE KEGEL

Contract the muscles around your anus, then around your vagina and into your urethra as though you were contracting these muscles toward your pubic bone. It will feel as though a wave were washing over your pelvic floor from your anus to your pubic bone. Slowly release the muscles from your urethra to anus as though the wave were releasing back to the shore. Start by simply contracting toward your pubic bone and releasing, and then see if you can slow down the motion, hold for a breath at the deepest contraction, and then release slowly.

BENEFITS OF KEGEL EXERCISES

Kegels help prevent urinary incontinence in late pregnancy and postpartum. Keeping your pelvic floor muscles in good tone will improve circulation and may prevent hemorrhoids. The perineal or pelvic floor muscles form a figure-eight pattern around the vagina and anus. You use these muscles automatically during love making and when you resist the urge to urinate. As you practice tightening and releasing these muscles, you will find that you can hold them in the contracted position for longer periods of time. You will also be better skilled at keeping them relaxed when you need to during the final stage of labor. We recommend that you perform fifty to one hundred Kegel exercises every day.

Yoga for Two

Take the time to move your body consciously and both you and your unborn baby will enjoy the benefits. Pregnancy affects every aspect of your body and yoga provides the opportunity for you to use your awareness to enliven healing and transformation in every tissue, organ, and cell. The flexibility that yoga cultivates in your body and mind will benefit you during your pregnancy, birth, and beyond.

Enliven Through Your Attention

- Place your hands on your belly a few times throughout the day and send loving thoughts to your unborn baby.
- Journal each day about your experiences.
- Early in your pregnancy, plant a tree or flowering bush to symbolize the growth of your baby in the womb. After your child is born, you can take care of the plant together.
- Read enchanting stories and heartfelt poetry aloud to your baby and listen to beautiful, relaxing music each day.
- Perform a daily oil massage on yourself before you bathe or shower.
- Diffuse an aroma while listening to music, while soaking in a tub, or while meditating to create the association between the fragrance and the relaxed state of awareness.
- Ensure that you have all six tastes available during your meals throughout the day.
- Choose to eat meals that are rich in color, aroma, and texture.
- Be mindful as you eat your meals. Eat at least one meal each week in silence with your full awareness.
- Practice meditation for twenty to thirty minutes twice daily.

• Pay attention to signals of stress you experience during the day and employ stress-reducing behaviors to minimize the harmful effects of stress on you and your unborn baby.

• Perform yoga postures with awareness on a regular basis, being gentle and respectful of your body.

CHAPTER 5

Weathering the Changes

Oh, ancient Spirit

That fire cannot burn, water cannot wet,

And wind cannot dry.

Your soul of unblemished joy has danced and cavorted

Across the vast ocean of consciousness

And stranded on my heart.

Beyond memories and anticipations,

The universe has conspired to create you.

Child of the universe, child of mine,

You are the eternal taking birth in time.

You are the Supreme Being

Creating a new world.

—DEEPAK CHOPRA

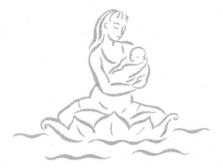

*P*regnancy is a time of dramatic change. Major transformations are taking place in your physiology as your unborn baby develops. Riding these waves of change can, at times, be challenging, and it is natural to experience emotional and physical ups and downs during pregnancy. Remember that although the ride may be bumpy at times, a smoother patch is right around the corner. Try not to compound your discomfort by being hard on yourself for feeling emotionally and physically unstable.

Although at other times of life you might be tempted to reach for a medication to soothe digestive upset, relieve muscular aches and pains, or overcome sleeping difficulties, most drugs are best avoided during pregnancy. Pregnancy, therefore, offers a great opportunity to experience the power of natural healing. The suggestions outlined in this chapter are offered as first-line approaches to common concerns during pregnancy. *They are not intended as a substitute for appropriate medical advice.* Incubating a new life is a sacred responsibility and, therefore, you do not want to take risks with your unborn baby's life. This means not taking pharmaceutical agents unnecessarily and not avoiding them when they are deemed essential.

A good channel of communication between you and your health care provider is an important component of a conscious pregnancy. We encourage you to discuss all options you are pursuing with your doctor or midwife throughout your pregnancy and labor. In most cases, your health advisor will support your use of gentle, natural approaches for common minor concerns that arise during pregnancy.

Morning Sickness

Almost three out of four women experience nausea during the first trimester of pregnancy, and about half of women who have nausea will be sick enough to vomit. Although this condition is most commonly referred to as morning sickness, the stomach queasiness in the beginning of pregnancy, which may last throughout the day, is often called *nausea and vom-*

iting in pregnancy (NVP). Although this condition has been carefully studied, it is still not certain what actually causes it. No pregnant woman welcomes the uncomfortable sensations of morning sickness, but it appears to actually have a positive impact. Women who experience morning sickness have a substantially lower risk of miscarriage than those who do not.

The nausea usually begins in the fifth week of gestation, peaks by eleven weeks, and typically subsides by the fifteenth or sixteenth week. Most women are no longer bothered by nausea during the second half of pregnancy, but for a small percentage of women, it lasts the entire forty weeks. On a scale of one to five, with five being most severe, the majority of women rate their symptoms of nausea at a level two or three; that is, enough to be really uncomfortable without being fully intolerable.

Several scientists have suggested that morning sickness provides a protective mechanism for the early embryo. The mother's sensitivity to many foods may keep her from ingesting substances that could potentially harm the unborn baby. The most common foods that pregnant women express aversion to during the first trimester are meat, poultry and fish, caffeine-containing beverages, and vegetables. From an evolutionary standpoint, avoidance by our ancestral mothers of potentially parasite-laden meat and phytochemically potent vegetables may have conferred protection for their vulnerable embryos. The tendency of modern mothers to crave fruits and fruit juices, grains, starches, sweets, and dairy may result from a selection process that increased the likelihood that

nutritional, safe, calorically rich foods became the nourishment of choice.

Studies have shown repeatedly that the rates of miscar-
riages and stillbirths are lower in women who have nausea.
Although some reports suggest that nausea is also associated
with fewer premature deliveries, higher birth weights,
reduced birth defects, and improved survival of infants, there
have been an equal number of contradictory reports that fail
to show any definite benefits related to these outcomes. We
do know that mothers with nausea eat less during their first
trimester and gain less weight. You might think that this
would be associated with smaller and less-healthy babies. As
it turns out, less weight gain in the first trimester results in an
increase in the size of the placenta, which supplies blood to
the developing fetus. As the nausea subsides, mothers
increase their food intake during the second and third
trimesters, their babies catch up, and the bigger placenta
ensures a healthy supply of food and oxygen. Similar patterns
of food intake have been reported in other mammals, including dogs, monkeys, and chimpanzees, supporting the idea that
NVP has a purpose.

Relieving the Upset

Knowing that nausea during the first part of pregnancy is protective may give you some consolation, but most mothers
would still be glad to see it subside. Medications used to treat

nausea in the past have notoriously bad reputations, and pharmaceutical companies have essentially abandoned efforts to find new drugs. This has opened the door to other, more natural, approaches.

Most women with nausea try a variety of techniques to quiet their queasy stomachs. A recent study from Canada found that the most common approaches that pregnant moms use to fight nausea are these:

Eating dry foods	Helpful or somewhat helpful in 64%
Lying down	Helpful or somewhat helpful in 59%
Clear or carbonated liquids	Helpful or somewhat helpful in 52%
Getting fresh air	Helpful or somewhat helpful in 40%
Mental concentration	Helpful or somewhat helpful in 33%

It is worth trying these simple approaches to reduce the nausea and vomiting of pregnancy. An expanded list of possible remedies includes ginger, other aromatic herbs, vitamin B_6, and acupressure, which we discuss in more detail below.

GINGER

The spicy rootstock of ginger has been prized around the world for thousands of years. With a number of unique natural chemicals, ginger is most often used to aid digestion and improve circulation. Studies from Denmark found that almost three out of four pregnant women received some relief of their nausea from ginger, without any limiting side effects.

Another study from Thailand reported that more than 87 percent of pregnant women using ginger had reduced nausea and vomiting (versus less than a third of those who took a placebo). Ginger appears to be safe for pregnancy. A Danish study found that ginger did not cause problems when given to pregnant rats at many times the dosage that a woman would normally take.

The easiest way to take ginger is to make a tea using 1 teaspoon of freshly grated gingerroot to 2 cups of hot water. Sweeten the tea with honey and sip it throughout the day. You can also chew on ½ teaspoon of grated gingerroot mixed with maple syrup when you are feeling nauseated.

OTHER AROMATIC HERBS

Aromatic herbs are used traditionally to stimulate digestion and have been promoted to relieve morning sickness. Peppermint, chamomile, and cinnamon teas can sometimes soothe an upset stomach, as can alfalfa. Try making a tea out of these herbs. Alternatively, try sucking on a clove bud.

VITAMIN B₆

Vitamin B_6 or pyridoxine was a component of the morning sickness drug Bendectin, which contained the antihistamine doxylamine. Despite the absence of convincing evidence of toxicity, Bendectin was taken off the market due to legal concerns. There is some evidence that B_6 alone may be helpful in reducing the nausea and vomiting of pregnancy at dosages of 25 milligrams every eight hours. Most prenatal vitamins contain between 20 milligrams and 50 milligrams of B_6. Although it is generally safe, B_6 can cause nerve toxicity at very high doses. Therefore, if you find B_6 helpful in reducing your morning sickness, limit your intake to not more than a total of 75 milligrams per day. Of interest, a study that attempted to correlate morning sickness with low blood B_6 levels could not find any relationship between vitamin B_6 status and the incidence or degree of morning sickness.

ACUPRESSURE

A number of studies have suggested that stimulation of the acupuncture point Pericardium 6 (P6) has an antinausea effect. This point, known as Neiguan, is located two finger

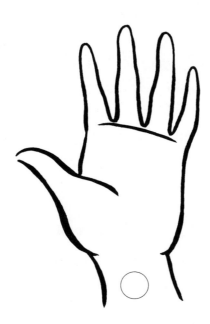

widths above the crease of your wrist in the middle of the palm side of your lower arm. You can stimulate the point by massaging it with your thumb or wearing an elastic band designed to stimulate the point. There is an inexpensive product on the market called the Sea-Band Wristband, which is commonly used by people prone to seasickness.

DIETARY ADJUSTMENTS

Try eating a few unsalted crackers or have a piece of toast upon arising in the morning. Light, easily digested foods are generally better tolerated than heavier ones. Eat protein-rich snacks and do your best to avoid greasy, fatty, or fried foods. Heed the messages your body is sending.

Other Digestive Disturbances

Your growing baby puts pressure on your digestive organs, commonly leading to indigestion, heartburn, bloating, and constipation. These minor but annoying digestive concerns are often amenable to simple, natural approaches.

HEARTBURN AND INDIGESTION

Heartburn and indigestion are frequent complaints during pregnancy, experienced most often during the last trimester. The growing womb squeezes the digestive tract, leading to congestion and bloating, and compresses the stomach, forcing acid into the esophagus and resulting in heartburn.

What Helps?

- Eat smaller meals throughout the day.
- Chew your food well. Don't swallow until it is fully liquefied.
- Reduce fatty and greasy foods.
- Eat or suck on slippery elm lozenges, an herb that can soothe an acidic stomach.
- Alfalfa, in the form of a pill, tea, or sprout, can help relieve indigestion and heartburn. Alfalfa contains eight different digestive enzymes and is rich in vitamins A, D, E, and K.
- Consume some milk or freshly made yogurt during the day.
- Drink fennel tea at the end of meals.
- Eat chewable calcium tablets to neutralize stomach acid.
- Chew on some orange peel after meals.
- Try dry-roasted coriander, cumin, or fennel seeds and chew on a pinch of them after each meal.
- Drink carbonated fluids.
- Use the herbs cardamom, cinnamon, and bay to dispel gas.

CONSTIPATION

Many women develop constipation during pregnancy. It is attributed in part to the hormone progesterone, which relaxes the smooth muscles of the gastrointestinal tract.

Pressure placed by the growing baby on the intestines also contributes to constipation.

What Helps?

- Drink lots of fresh water and juices.
- Exercise daily.
- Increase your intake of fresh fruits, salads, and vegetables.
- Include in your diet foods rich in fiber.
- Consider taking alfalfa, which may help relieve constipation.
- Eat several prunes and raisins each day.

HEMORRHOIDS

Due to the buildup of abdominal pressure throughout pregnancy, hemorrhoids are a common concern. With the straining that occurs during labor, they often worsen after birth. Pressure in the belly and pelvis impedes the return of blood supply, causing rectal blood vessels to dilate. Also, increased levels of progesterone during pregnancy relax smooth muscles, slowing blood flow through the veins.

What Helps?

- Exercise regularly to improve circulation and muscle tone.

- Drink plenty of fluids.
- Eat more fiber-rich foods to reduce constipation and the need for forceful evacuation.
- Consider vitamin E, which may be helpful in maintaining elasticity in the veins.
- Use fresh garlic, which also may be helpful in retaining vein elasticity.
- Reduce spicy foods.
- Support healthy blood vessels with the natural chemicals in berries and cherries.
- Sip nettle tea throughout the day—it is great for vein elasticity.
- Avoid sitting for long periods of time.
- Use witch hazel for pain or itching hemorrhoids. Presoaked pads are available at pharmacies. You can apply witch hazel directly to your bottom or soak an ice pack in witch hazel and apply it.
- Try a comfrey compress on your bottom by brewing some leaves and soaking a clean washcloth in the decoction. (Comfrey is known for its healing and pain-relieving qualities.)
- Do Kegel exercises throughout the day to increase circulation in the perineum.

INSOMNIA

Restless sleep is almost universal during pregnancy, particularly during the last trimester.

What Helps?

- Exercise each day.
- Wind down intense mental activity at least one hour before your regular bedtime.
- Perform a self-massage, followed by a warm aroma bath with lavender or vanilla.
- Drink a cup of chamomile tea before bed.
- Try a glass of warm milk with cardamom, nutmeg, or a pinch of saffron before bed.
- Listen to relaxing music.
- Place pillows under your belly and between your legs. A body pillow works great at the end of pregnancy.

NASAL CONGESTION

More than one in five pregnant women complain of nasal congestion, which is often most disturbing in the evening hours and may interfere with sleep. The exact cause of this problem is not clear. Nasal congestion in pregnancy does not seem to be an allergic reaction and does not respond to the usual medications. Circulating hormones may contribute to the swelling of mucous membranes inside the nose, resulting in congestion and a runny nose.

What Helps?

- Drink plenty of fluids.
- Get plenty of fresh air.

- Try a vaporizer or humidifier.
- Use a neti pot. Add some warm salt water to the pot and administer to the nasal passages. Follow this by applying some sesame oil or ghee to your nose.

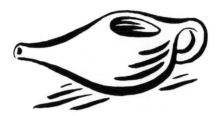

- Try the Breathing Easy nasal patches when you sleep or lie down. These are available in most pharmacies.

LEG CRAMPS

It is not unusual to experience leg cramps as your body attempts to adjust to the rapid physical and hormonal changes of pregnancy. Studies have shown that almost half of all pregnant woman experience leg cramps, most often in the second half of pregnancy. Although they can occur throughout the day, they are most common and most severe at night.

What Helps?

- Exercise every day.
- Elevate your legs frequently during the day.

- Massage your calves and thighs with oil on a daily basis.
- Ensure that you are receiving abundant calcium and magnesium in your diet. Good natural calcium sources are dark leafy greens, kelp, cheese, yogurt, soy milk, nuts, and fruits. Magnesium-rich foods include nuts, legumes, whole-grain cereals, dark green vegetables, soybeans, and seafood.
- Discuss with your health provider the need for magnesium supplementation.
- Sip raspberry leaf or nettle tea.
- Include vitamin E–rich foods such as wheat germ, spinach, and dried fruit in your diet.
- To relieve leg cramps as they occur, stretch your calf muscle by bending your foot toward your head and rotating your ankle.
- Apply warm compresses to the cramped area.

BACKACHE

As pregnancy progresses, your body secretes chemicals that loosen the joints and ligaments in preparation for birth. The increased weight of your growing baby along with the laxity of the ligaments may cause your back to ache.

What Helps?

- Exercise daily.
- Avoid heavy lifting and always bend your knees when lifting objects below your waist.

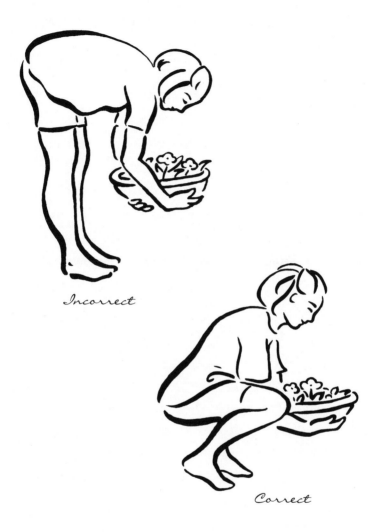

Incorrect

Correct

- Practice yoga.
- Relax in a warm aroma bath.
- Receive back massages to relax and release tight muscles.
- Take time out to rest a little while each day.
- Apply warm heat to your back.

143

- Ensure adequate calcium and magnesium in your diet.
- Drink plenty of fluids.
- Sleep with pillows under your knees and use pillows to support your back and growing belly.

MOOD SWINGS

Fluctuating moods are common during pregnancy. There are a lot of changes taking place in your body, which affect your emotions. Be gentle with yourself and know that some emotional turbulence is normal. Having a baby will change your life, and some anxiety over these changes is healthy.

What Helps?

- Meditate regularly.
- Practice yoga.
- Exercise daily.
- Take time to relax by listening to soothing music or guided visualizations.
- Take naps when you are tired.
- Soak in a warm aroma bath.
- Honor the changes you are experiencing and find ways to nurture yourself.
- Communicate your needs and concerns to your family and your social support network.

- Journal about your feelings each day.
- Increase your energy by eating high-protein snacks.
- Drink plenty of fluids.
- Sip chamomile or raspberry leaf tea.
- If anxiety or depression is interfering with your daily life, be sure to promptly communicate your concerns to your health care provider.

SWELLING

Minor swelling of the hands, ankles, and feet is common during the final weeks of pregnancy. The hormonal changes associated with pregnancy may result in fluid retention, and your enlarging womb places pressure on the large veins that return blood to the heart.

What Helps?

- Rest with your feet elevated.
- Exercise daily.
- Avoid tight-fitting clothes.
- Avoid sitting for long periods of time, particularly with your knees bent and your feet on the floor.
- Massage your feet, legs, arms, and hands.
- Soak your feet in a tub.
- Limit your intake of salty foods such as potato chips and pretzels.

If swelling becomes excessive, call your health care provider.

URINARY TRACT INFECTIONS

Urinary tract infections (UTI) are not uncommon during pregnancy. The growing uterus compresses the bladder, which can inhibit complete emptying. When urine stagnates in the bladder, it is easier for bacteria to grow. The composition of urine becomes less acidic during pregnancy and contains higher levels of hormones, predisposing you to bacterial infections. Untreated UTIs are potentially dangerous for both the mother and the fetus.

What Helps?

- Drink plenty of fluids.
- Drink cranberry juice, which has been shown to reduce the adherence of bacteria to the bladder lining.
- Urinate frequently.
- Wipe yourself from front to back to reduce the risk of introducing bacteria into the bladder.
- Use cotton underwear. Cotton breathes easier than other materials.
- If you have any burning or discomfort during urination, call your health care provider.

When to Call Your Health Care Advisor

An open channel of communication between you and your health care provider is an important component of a conscious pregnancy. You should have a low threshold for calling your doctor or midwife, as it is better to be overly cautious and learn that your concern is a normal variation, than to be dismissive of a symptom that may be an important warning signal. The following are certain signs and symptoms that should be brought to the immediate attention of your health care provider:

- vaginal bleeding
- severe or persistent abdominal pain or cramping
- severe headaches or blurred vision
- shortness of breath or chest pain
- swelling of your ankles, hands, or face
- reduced urine output
- burning or discomfort during urination
- fever of 101° Fahrenheit or higher
- fluid leaking from your vagina
- an increased or foul-smelling vaginal discharge
- a decrease in fetal movements
- marked gain in weight
- an increase in pelvic pressure before thirty-five weeks of gestation

- contractions occurring more than four times per hour
- any other symptom that worries you or seems abnormal.

Exercise

ENVISIONING YOUR BODY

Have your journal, some colored markers, and a pen nearby.

Start by closing your eyes for a few minutes and connect to your body and breath. Allow your awareness to journey through your body from the top of your head to your toes. Notice where you feel tight and where you feel open. Feel where your breath most easily moves. Stay with your breath for a few moments, inhaling and exhaling. Feel each breath bringing you nourishment and energy.

As you sit, quietly feel how your belly is becoming rounder and fuller. Bring your awareness to your belly and feel the sensations there. Feel your breath in your belly and acknowledge how it feels to have your belly becoming rounder and your body becoming fuller. Feel how your baby is being held and cradled safely inside of your womb. Notice what it feels like to have a baby growing inside your belly. Feel your breath rising and falling within you and notice your feelings about your body changing in shape and size.

As you continue to feel your breath, allow your awareness to flow to your genitals and your breasts. Notice how you feel about yourself as a woman and how you feel about your sexuality. With your next breath acknowledge yourself as the mother of this tiny baby. Feel your connection to all mothers and to all women. Take as much time as you need to explore your sensations and feelings. When you feel complete and ready, slowly open your eyes.

Now retrieve your colored markers and draw a picture of your pregnant body. For example, you might want to mark where you feel tight and where you feel open in your body. Pick a color to express how you are feeling in your belly and inside your womb. Allow the picture to describe what you experience. Let go of the need to be a great artist and have fun.

Take some time to journal about your picture and your feelings. Allow your thoughts to flow freely without holding back anything. Release any judgment or criticism about your feelings or sensations. Honor yourself completely.

Enliven Through Your Attention

• Place your hands on your belly a few times throughout the day and send loving thoughts to your unborn baby.

• Journal each day about your experiences.

• Early in your pregnancy, plant a tree or flowering bush to symbolize the growth of your baby in the womb. After your child is born, you can take care of the plant together.

• Read enchanting stories and heartfelt poetry aloud to your baby and listen to beautiful, relaxing music each day.

• Perform a daily oil massage on yourself before you bathe or shower.

• Diffuse an aroma while listening to music, while soaking in a tub, or while meditating to create the association between the fragrance and the relaxed state of awareness.

• Ensure that you have all six tastes available during your meals throughout the day.

• Choose to eat meals that are rich in color, aroma, and texture.

• Be mindful as you eat your meals. Eat at least one meal each week in silence with your full awareness.

• Practice meditation for twenty to thirty minutes twice daily.

• Pay attention to signals of stress that you experience during the day and employ stress-reducing behaviors to minimize the harmful effects of stress on you and your unborn baby.

• Perform yoga postures with awareness on a regular basis, being gentle and respectful of your body.

• Embrace your pregnancy as an opportunity to experience more natural healing approaches to common minor health concerns.

• Whenever an uncomfortable symptom arises, go through a mental checklist to ensure that you are taking time to relax, eating properly, drinking enough fluids, and exercising regularly.

• Develop an open line of communication with your health care provider and have a low threshold for calling about any emotional or physical concern that may arise.

CHAPTER 6

Partners in Love

You are the seed of enchanted forests of mystical realms.

Together we will nurture our desires

In the sacred corridors of our souls.

And one day these desires will burst into flame,

And in the burnished glow,

and sudden splendor of love,

We will dream a new world of reality

From the purity of our hearts.

—DEEPAK CHOPRA

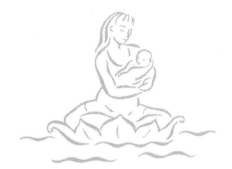

*E*ach human being is woven from the genetic and behavioral threads of his or her parents. The relationship patterns that your child is exposed to, before and after birth, shape her mental and physical well-being. Whether you and your partner create a traditional nuclear family or choose to explore one of the other modern variations in child rearing, developing your communication skills is essential to a healthy and nourishing emotional life.

Pregnancy is a landmark event in a couple's relationship. When two people make the choice to parent a child, both

partners assume a new level of responsibility. In every relationship, there are times when needs and expectations
bring to the surface underlying emotional issues. Almost all
psychological disciplines acknowledge the presence of an
inner emotional child in most chronologically adult human
beings. When you create a baby, you will have another
inner child fully dependent upon you to meet her needs.
For your benefit and the benefit of your family, we encourage you to use your pregnancy as an opportunity to heal
unresolved emotional issues and improve your communication skills.

Pregnancy is a time of dynamic transformation with
numerous physical and emotional challenges. It is normal
and natural for parents to encounter a wide range of emotions
during pregnancy. As mothers and fathers anticipate how a
new baby will change their lives, it is common to feel happiness as well as apprehension. Acknowledging, accepting, and
embracing this ambivalence is important, because anything
we resist persists, and eventually creates distress. Many years
ago, Freud recognized that the inability to tolerate ambivalence was the root of neurosis. By recognizing and accepting
the diverse feelings we have without judgment, we are better
able to respond to challenges in ways that reflect our highest
values.

In addition to emotions of excitement, enthusiasm, and
joy that usually predominate, it is not uncommon for a pregnant woman to experience feelings of anxiety, trepidation,
and uneasiness. Among other issues, a mom-to-be may feel

concerned about her rapidly changing body shape, her wider-than-usual mood fluctuations, her ability to be a good parent, and changes in her career path. The father-to-be may be uneasy about losing his partner's attention, her changing sexual drive, his competence as a parent, and the financial costs of raising a child.

Acknowledging and developing the skills to express these darker emotions helps you free up creative energy that can otherwise be trapped in the denial of these completely normal feelings. We frequently see pregnant couples at the Chopra Center who are troubled by ambivalent feelings they have been afraid to express. When they learn that most people share these emotions, and that they are not destined to be poor parents just because they have doubts or fears, a tremendous weight is removed from their hearts and their delight in the pregnancy is able to shine through.

Take a couple of minutes now to consider the various feelings, concerns, and questions you have about becoming a parent and express them in your journal.

Like the imagined monster in the closet that generates anxiety in the child who is carried away by her worst fears, your unspoken concerns are often the ones that generate the most distressing emotions. Begin by acknowledging them to yourself, and then use your best communication skills to express your concerns to your partner. A couple that participated in one of our recent workshops found tremendous relief by performing this simple exercise.

Mom's Responses

COMFORTABLE FEELINGS/ISSUES

  UNCOMFORTABLE FEELINGS/ISSUES

I'm feeling really excited about becoming a mother.

  I'm conflicted about how much time I should take off from work.

I love my big breasts.

  I am tired of this morning sickness.

I'm feeling more connected to my older sister who has two children.

  Will everything go okay with my labor and birth?

I like focusing on eating healthy foods.

  Am I gaining too much weight?

Dad's Responses

COMFORTABLE FEELINGS/ISSUES

  UNCOMFORTABLE FEELINGS/ISSUES

I can't wait to be a parent and share my love.

  I'm concerned that our small house will not be big enough for my family.

I feel more connected than ever with my wife.

  I feel pressure about the cost of raising a family.

My life seems to have more purpose as I think about my new family.

  Will my wife and I have any time alone together after the baby's here?

My wife seems gentler and more emotionally available.

  Although my wife's been cuddly, she hasn't had much interest in sex.

When this couple had the opportunity to express their concerns in a safe and nonjudgmental exchange, each partner felt relief and deeper intimacy. When hearing the concerns of your partner, it is best to simply acknowledge them without attempting to "solve" the other person's problem. Simply saying, "I can understand how you might have that concern," or "Thanks for sharing your concerns with me," is usually more effective than trying to convince the other person that their anxieties are unnecessary. Remember, ambivalence is a healthy aspect of human emotions. Acknowledging the dark side does not negate the positive aspects.

Waging Peace

We all prefer environments that exude peace and harmony. Most of us do not willingly go into a battle zone. An unborn baby is aware of her environment as she grows inside the womb and responds to her mother's feeling of comfort or agitation. The story of the family as told through both words and feelings is learned by the unborn baby long before birth. Put your attention on learning to heal upsets with your partner before your child arrives. Open your heart and clear any toxic emotions that may be residing there. Make your home a garden of peace so your baby will feel safe and cherished both before and after her first breath is taken. Allow your baby's beginning to be innocent, harmonious, and filled with wonder. Healthy, loving communication is its own reward in every relationship. Using your pregnancy as a catalyst to enhance a deeper connection between you and your partner will reap benefits for all the members of your family.

The ABCs of Emotion

Emotions engage both your mind and body. Emotions are distinguished from other thoughts by the accompaniment of physical sensations. Emotions are primary mind-body experiences. If you hear that a company in your town is going out of business, it may transiently catch your interest. If it is the company that you or your spouse is employed by, it is likely that the information in your mind will be accompanied by potent sensations in your body. We call these sensations feelings because we actually feel them in our physical body. When we use language to characterize our emotions such as, "I felt like I was kicked in the stomach," or "I felt my heart was breaking," our words are describing the sensations generated in our bodies.

Although our emotions come in many different flavors, they ultimately boil down to two primary feelings: comfort and discomfort. As a result of what you see and hear in your world, your body interprets the experience as being either nourishing or threatening. All feelings are reducible to comfort or discomfort, pleasure or pain, happiness or sadness, or as novelist Tom Robbins once said, "Yum or yuck." Whether you are consciously aware of it or not, every choice you make is based upon your expectation that the choice will bring you greater comfort and less discomfort. Every decision you make, from your order at a restaurant, to the style of shoes you buy, to the job you take, is based upon the expectation that your choice will result in greater comfort or less discomfort. Sometimes we are willing to endure immediate discomfort for the expectation of longer-term comfort, such as when we exercise, undergo a medical procedure, or forgo dessert; but even these choices are ultimately based on the belief that the anticipated long-term pleasure outweighs the short-term pain.

Given the same circumstance or situation, different people have different emotional reactions. If you are a pure vegetarian, being served a helping of Grandma's meatloaf will not elicit the pleasurable sensations that a meat eater experiences. Your teenager may experience intense pleasure listening to hip-hop music while it may give you a headache. Some people revel in the exhilaration of a roller-coaster ride, while for others it would be a nightmare. It is not the inherent experience that generates feelings of comfort or discomfort; rather, it is your interpretation of the experience.

Why does one person enjoy a scary horror movie while another relishes a romantic comedy? The answer boils down to a simple principle that is obvious when you observe children. What you will soon discover when your baby is born is that *feelings derive from needs*. When a child gets what she wants when she wants it, she feels comfortable. When she does not get what she wants, or gets what she doesn't want (like a bath or an early bedtime), she feels uncomfortable. Positive emotions arise when we feel that our needs are being met. Negative emotions arise when we feel our needs are not being met.

Conscious Communication

The more successful you are in meeting your needs, the more likely you are to spend time in states of emotional comfort. When it comes to interpersonal needs—the needs we have in relation to the people in our lives—communication is the most important determinant of need fulfillment. If you are skilled at communicating your needs, you are more likely to see them satisfied. Unfortunately, most people are not masters at communicating their needs.

It is common for people to hold the idea that what they require is so obvious that the other person should simply "know" what they want. Many have an unspoken expectation that "If you really love me, you should be able to read my heart and mind, and give me what I need without me having to ask for it." Most children actually enjoyed a period of time when this was the case. An infant child cries and an attentive mother urgently attempts to diagnose the need and fulfill it: "Is she cold? Is she hungry? Does she need her diaper changed? Is she tired and needs a nap?" As people mature emotionally, they learn to meet more of their own needs and, ideally, learn to communicate effectively so others are able to understand and meet their needs. Because most people have never received formal education in communication, we would like to review a simple process that we have found to be very helpful. Drawing upon the work of psychologist Marshall Rosenberg, this process of conscious communication avoids wasting emotional energy on labels and judgments, and focuses on successful strategies to increase comfort and decrease distress.

There are five key questions that we encourage you to address whenever emotional turbulence is activated in your body/mind: What is occurring to trigger my emotions? What emotions are arising within me? What do I need that I am not receiving? What am I getting out of *not* having my needs met? What am I really asking for?

We'll review these questions one at a time in more detail.

WHAT IS OCCURRING TO TRIGGER MY EMOTIONS?

Situations in the present frequently remind us of similar circumstances from the past, evoking memories and feelings that may have little to do with what is actually occurring now. For example, you may be driving on a trip with your partner who has fallen silent. This triggers a memory of your parents not talking to each other for days at a time. As a result you say to your partner, "What are you angry about? Why are you being so cold to me?" Your partner is surprised and responds, "I was just thinking about how we can arrange the baby's room so it won't feel too crowded."

It is very useful to separate out what you are seeing and hearing from your interpretation. In this example, after your partner did not speak for ten minutes, you interpreted this silence as anger or withholding. Begin to notice how often you substitute your *interpretations* for your *observations*. Your doctor does not return your call within an hour and you label him as uncaring. Your sister arrives fifteen minutes after the time you were scheduled to meet for lunch and you judge her as selfish and narcissistic. Your partner talks to another person at a party and you label it as flirting. Whether your analysis is accurate or not, replacing your description of what is occurring with your interpretation rarely increases the likelihood that you will get your needs met.

On some level, judgment always involves some rejection. People respond to this subtle sense of rejection and become less willing and able to give you what you need. Have the intention to avoid judging and see how you waste less time in states of emotional turbulence.

WHAT EMOTIONS ARE ARISING WITHIN ME?

As a consequence of something you saw or heard, emotions are activated. Develop an expanded vocabulary of your emotions and you will find that uncomfortable feelings dissipate much more quickly. If you are visiting a foreign land and have a limited grasp of the native language, you become frustrated in your efforts to communicate your needs. Since most people have limited emotional vocabularies, they compound their unhappiness by their inability to express what is happening inside them.

In his insightful book *Nonviolent Communication*, Dr. Rosenberg points out that certain words we use to express our feelings increase our sense of victimization, and are therefore better avoided. When you say, "I feel . . . abandoned . . . neglected . . . rejected . . . abused . . . unappreciated . . ." or "manipulated," you are holding other people accountable for your emotions and setting up a situation where someone else has to change in order for you to feel better. If you are uncomfortable because you believe someone is manipulating you, they must stop their behavior in order for you to feel better. If you are waiting for someone else to change in order for you to feel more comfortable, we hope you have a large reservoir of patience.

Rather than relinquishing your power to external circumstances, we encourage you to own your feelings, and use language that reduces interpretation and conveys your willingness to accept responsibility. Rather than saying, "When I saw you flirting, I felt abandoned by you," try "When I saw you talking to that person, I felt anxious, jealous, and irritable." Using language that conveys your responsibility for your feelings will reduce the likelihood that your partner will move into a reactive emotional mode, and increases the probability that you will get your needs met.

Practice expanding your emotional vocabulary so you do

not resort to the language of victimization. An alphabetical listing of suggested empowering words is presented below.

Anxious	Helpless	Pessimistic
Bitter	Invisible	Queasy
Confused	Jealous	Resentful
Discouraged	Lonely	Sorry
Empty	Mad	Tired
Frustrated	Nauseated	Uneasy
Guilty	Obstinate	Withdrawn

WHAT DO I NEED THAT I AM NOT RECEIVING?

If you are experiencing uncomfortable emotions, it is because you have a need that is not being met. If you are not clear about what that need is, it is unlikely that someone else will be able to figure it out for you. Become clear about what you seek and you will substantially increase your chances of getting it.

Needs can be seen from a variety of perspectives. According to Ayurveda, we have four basic needs. We have a need for material comforts, known as *Artha*; we need love and connection, known as *Kama*; we need a sense of purpose in life, known as *Dharma*; and we need spiritual awakening, known as *Moksha*, or liberation. Whenever you feel emotionally upset, one of these needs is being threatened.

Human beings need to maintain healthy ego boundaries. This means having the freedom and personal power to say "no" when it is in your highest interest. When your boundaries are healthy, you allow energy and information to move into your life when you believe it is nourishing but maintain appropriate defenses when an encounter carries potentially toxic consequences. Boundaries crossed without permission create emotional pain.

When you are in the midst of emotional turbulence, see if you can identify what you need that you are not getting or how your boundary was crossed without your consent. Then, see if there are other unspoken issues that are subconsciously sabotaging your ability to meet your needs. This brings us to the next question.

WHAT AM I GETTING OUT OF *NOT* HAVING MY OBVIOUS NEEDS MET?

When we participate in situations that generate emotional conflict or turbulence, there is usually another conversation taking place within us at a deeper level of awareness. This realm of consciousness, commonly referred to as the shadow, stirs up strong feelings because these deeper needs may be in conflict with those on the surface. Perhaps you believe that intense emotions are necessary to keep a relationship alive and need conflict to generate the intensity. Perhaps you need more drama in your primary relationship because your own life is lacking in passion. Perhaps your need for control or your need to be "right" exceeds your need for harmony. Perhaps, even as you consciously state your desire for greater intimacy, you create conflict because you are afraid of the vulnerability that the intimacy requires.

If you find yourself in a pattern of recurrent conflict with your partner, ask yourself what you might be getting out of the clashes. See if the current situation is reminiscent of earlier intimate relationships. Ask yourself if there are other issues, unrelated to the conflict, seeking expression. Quiet your mind, ask the questions, and see if any insight dawns.

WHAT AM I REALLY ASKING FOR?

Your chances of meeting your needs will be substantially enhanced if you formulate a request and ask for what you want. It is not uncommon to substitute a demand for a request, but outside the military this diminishes rather than increases the likelihood that your needs will be met. Making a request requires a willingness to be vulnerable, because there is always the possibility of hearing that dread word "No." However, asking for a specific behavior that the person is capable of performing increases the likelihood that you'll get what you need.

Don't waste your energy asking for someone to think, believe, or feel a certain way. Rather than saying, "I just need for you to feel how much I am hurting," try "Can you put your arms around me?" Rather than saying, "I need for you to spend more time with me," try asking, "Can we meet for lunch tomorrow?" The more specific you make your request, the more likely your need will be met and your feelings will change from uncomfortable to comfortable.

You have an appointment with your obstetrician and ask your husband to meet you there. He gets stuck in traffic and arrives twenty minutes after your visit has started. You feel upset. Consider the following two scenarios of how you might express yourself as you are leaving the doctor's office.

SCENARIO #1   SCENARIO #2

WHAT IS OCCURRING TO TRIGGER MY EMOTIONS?

"I can't believe you were late. You're so inconsiderate. Knowing you, you'll probably miss the birth."

"I told you the appointment started at 10:30 and you arrived at 10:50."

WHAT EMOTIONS ARE ARISING WITHIN ME?

"When you weren't there at the start of my appointment, I felt abandoned by you. You're never there when I need you."

"When you weren't there at the start of my appointment, I felt anxious and insecure."

WHAT DO I NEED THAT I AM NOT RECEIVING?

"You should know what I need. I need what every pregnant woman would need. I need you to be there for me."

"I need to feel that this baby is a high priority for you. I need for you to hear what the doctor says so we can discuss it. I need to feel your support throughout the pregnancy."

SCENARIO #1	SCENARIO #2

WHAT AM I GETTING OUT OF NOT HAVING MY NEEDS MET?

"I'm not getting anything out of this argument. If you were a good husband you would be there by my side."	"Perhaps I need to blow off steam because I feel nervous and out of control in medical environments. Directing my frustration at my husband gives me a sense of control."

WHAT AM I REALLY ASKING FOR?

"You need to be on time and make me feel safe if we're going to make a family together."	"I feel nervous when I'm at the doctor's office without you. Can you promise me that at the next appointment you will arrive on time?"

Learning to communicate your needs more consciously increases the probability that your needs will be met. It doesn't mean that you will get everything that you want, but improving communication skills will improve the chances of getting more of what you seek. When both parties are committed to honestly expressing needs in ways that make it possible for them to be fulfilled, everyone wins.

Dealing with Upsets

Even with the best communication skills, normal, healthy people get upset. There will be frequent times when your needs are not met exactly as you would choose and your ego boundaries are crossed without your permission. It is unrealistic to expect that you will completely avoid emotional turbulence, but it is realistic to expect that you can regain your emotional center more quickly by using tools to digest emotionally charged experiences. Keeping the emotional body clear is essential to good health. People tend to hold on to emotional hurts, betrayals, and disappointments, because they have not been taught effective ways to deal with them. As a result of trying to suppress the pain associated with emotional wounding, many do not experience the joy and vitality they would like.

Undigested emotions, like undigested food, result in the accumulation of toxicity in our physiology. We offer seven steps for releasing emotional toxicity.

1. Take *responsibility* for what you are feeling. When you find yourself reacting emotionally to other people, it is usually because they are reflecting some quality that you have not fully acknowledged about your own nature. Accept responsibility for your emotions and you will cease to be a bundle of conditioned reflexes, which makes you vulnerable to

the opinions of every person you encounter. When you find yourself in a reactive mode with someone, ask the question "What can I learn about myself from this experience?" See if you can identify in the other person a quality you feel upset about, which you have been denying in yourself. This is the Mirror of Relationships principle: "Those we love and those we hate are both mirrors of ourselves."

2. Identify the emotion. "I feel_____." It may be *angry, sad, hurt, jealous, lonely,* etc. As clearly as possible, define and describe what you are feeling, avoiding language that encourages a sense of victimization.

3. Witness the feeling in your body. Emotions are thoughts associated with physical sensations. Upsetting thoughts trigger uncomfortable bodily reactions. The chemistry associated with emotions has a life of its own that must be acknowledged before the emotion can be processed further. Just observe the feeling, allowing your attention to embrace the sensation. By simply experiencing the physical sensations, you'll find the charge of the emotion dissipates.

4. Express your emotions privately to yourself. Write about your feelings in a journal you keep just for this purpose. Use the five questions elaborated above to explore the meaning of the emotional upset. Allow memories of similar situations to come to the surface and write about them, too. Use language that accurately conveys what you are feeling.

Allow yourself to express all that you need to about the situation.

5. Release the emotion through some ritual. Physical movement is usually best for this. Go for a walk, dance, swim, or perform yoga with deep-breathing exercises. Allow your body to discharge the emotional tension from your physiology.

6. Share the emotion with the person involved in the situation once you feel more centered. If you have gone through steps 1 through 5, it should be possible to share your feelings without casting blame, expecting pity, or trying to make the other person feel guilty.

7. Rejuvenate! If you've gone through steps 1 through 6, you deserve to be rewarded—so reward yourself for your good work. Do something nice for yourself. Get a massage, listen to music, buy yourself a present, eat a delicious meal—nourish yourself.

Conscious Listening

One of the most important communication skills you can develop is that of conscious listening. Often when someone shares a concern, the other person feels the need to fix the problem. In the attempt to be helpful, a response may be formulated even before the issue has been fully communicated. More often than not, the person is not seeking suggestions on how to fix the problem as much as simply needing to be heard. Listening attentively to another's concerns, instead of immediately trying to make it better, cultivates feelings of being understood and facilitates resolution of the problem. See if you can agree to the following "rules of engagement" with your partner.

• We take turns being the one who expresses and the one who listens.

• When I am the expresser, I use language such as "I feel . . ." rather than "You made me feel . . ."

• As the listener, I demonstrate my attention through my expressions and gestures and by repeating what I have heard from you.

• We make the commitment to have regular conscious communication sessions with each other. We will reward each other for successful listening sessions—going for walks, taking a bubble bath together, going out for romantic dinners, giving each other massages, making love.

Enliven Through Your Attention

• Place your hands on your belly a few times throughout the day and send loving thoughts to your unborn baby.

• Journal each day about your experiences.

- Early in your pregnancy, plant a tree or flowering bush to symbolize the growth of your baby in the womb. After your child is born, you can take care of the plant together.

- Read enchanting stories and heartfelt poetry aloud to your baby and listen to beautiful, relaxing music each day.

- Perform a daily oil massage on yourself before you bathe or shower.

- Diffuse an aroma while listening to music, while soaking in a tub, or while meditating to create the association between the fragrance and the relaxed state of awareness.

- Ensure that you have all six tastes available during your meals throughout the day.

- Choose to eat meals that are rich in color, aroma, and texture.

- Be mindful as you eat your meals. Eat at least one meal each week in silence with your full awareness.

- Practice meditation for twenty to thirty minutes twice daily.

- Pay attention to signals of stress that you experience during the day and employ stress-reducing behaviors to minimize the harmful effects of stress on you and your unborn baby.

- Perform yoga postures with awareness on a regular basis, being gentle and respectful of your body.

- Embrace your pregnancy as an opportunity to experience more natural healing approaches to common minor health concerns.

- Whenever an uncomfortable symptom arises, go through

a mental checklist to ensure that you are taking time to re-lax, eating properly, drinking enough fluids, and exercising regularly.

• Develop an open line of communication with your health care provider and have a low threshold for calling about any emotional or physical concern that may arise.

• Commit to improving your conscious communication skills. When you are feeling upset, determine what you really need and ask for the behavior that will fulfill your need.

• Practice the seven steps for emotional clearing when you are experiencing emotional turbulence. Notice how empower-ing the process can be when you take responsibility for your feelings.

• Whenever you are finding it difficult to communicate with your partner about your feelings, create the opportunity to prac-tice conscious listening.

CHAPTER 7

The Birthing Journey

Our deepest fear is not that we are inadequate.

Our deepest fear is that we are powerful beyond measure.

It is our light, not our darkness, that most frightens us. . . .

And as we let our own light shine,

We unconsciously give other people

Permission to do the same.

As we are liberated from our own fear,

Our presence automatically liberates others.

—MARIANNE WILLIAMSON

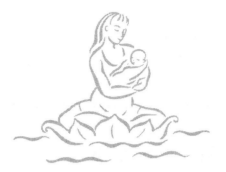

*W*e believe that pregnancy and birth are natural processes and that whenever possible, less medical intervention is preferable to more. We also recognize and support the reality that each birth is a very personal event, reflecting the perceptions, beliefs, experiences, and choices of the pregnant mom. Our bottom line is that the ultimate measurement of a successful pregnancy and birth is not how much or how little technological intervention is brought to bear; rather, it is a birth that results in the healthiest possible baby and mom.

You have spent the past nine months preparing for this

momentous event. Your regular meditation practice has established your connection to the essence of your being— your spirit that is beyond time and space. Yoga has helped you develop flexibility in both your mind and body. You have used soothing aromas to create the association between your sense of smell and relaxation. Your daily massage has ensured that your tissues are lubricated and pliable. You have worked with your breath and experienced how it can bring you into a deep place of inner quietness. You are prepared in your body, mind, and spirit to birth your baby.

Birthing a baby is probably the most powerful physical and emotional experience of a woman's life. After nine months of development, your unborn baby is ready to leave the loving cocoon of your womb and enter the world through your body. A conscious birth recognizes and honors the spiritual significance of bringing this being into the world. Working in consort with the powerful forces of nature, you give birth to your baby.

Conception, pregnancy, and childbirth are natural events, which express life's creative power on physical, emotional, and spiritual levels. Your and your family's perceptions, interpretations, and expectations play an important role in achieving a successful birthing experience. We believe you should be empowered with knowledge that enables you to make informed choices regarding the labor and birth of your baby.

Understanding life as an expression of a deeper non-local field of intelligence has profound effects on the way in which you experience yourself and others. Living your life from a consciousness-based perspective implies that you view every aspect of your life as meaningful, even sacred. A consciousness-based approach applied to pregnancy and birth means that the vision of your baby-to-be encompasses physical, emotional, and spiritual domains.

Awaken to the beauty and power inside your body. Pregnancy and labor are times to turn within. They are times of profound transition and transformation. While traveling this

Whatever your powerful mind believes will come to pass.

—PARAMHANSA YOGANANDA

journey you are required to embrace fear and trepidation along with wisdom and strength. Each stage of labor brings growth and change.

Exploring Your Fears

As a woman, you have been accumulating ideas about birthing since your childhood. You may have observed your mother pregnant with a younger sibling and her changing body and mind. You probably heard stories about labor and birth and may have seen movies of women in labor. You may have been present at the birth of a younger sibling, niece, or nephew.

At time these stories and images may have portrayed the birthing process as agonizing. If you have been exposed to frightening birthing stories, you may fear that labor will cause unbearable pain and be terrified at the thought of losing control. If these are the deep-rooted messages you have accepted, you may think of labor as an experience you need to be rescued from rather than one that empowers you. Fear of pain has resulted in many women losing sight of birth as normal and natural, and of themselves as powerful and capable. Labor is an opportunity for women to learn about themselves and discover the strength and wisdom inherent in their bodies.

Facing Your Fears

Bringing unconscious fears out into the open is the best way to dissipate the influence they have over you. Like the boogeyman you may have imagined living in your closet as a child, most fears lose their power when exposed to the light of awareness. We encourage you to perform the following exercise to become more aware of the positive and negative thoughts, words, and images about labor and birth that dwell within your mind. Becoming more aware of your inner conversation about birthing will enable you to make more conscious choices that accurately reflect your values.

Exercise

Sit for a few minutes with your eyes closed and envision the process of giving birth to your baby. Imagine the process from the first contractions to holding your baby in your arms.

Now, focus on your concerns. What are you afraid of with regard to labor and birth? On a sheet of paper write down the fearful words that come to mind.

Once you have listed these words describing your anxiety, take a few moments to create a separate list describing the feelings these expressions generate within your body (*these fearful words generate the following emotions and sensations within me*).

Now, again, close your eyes and envision your labor and birth. This time focus on your positive expectations. Make a list of the empowering words that come into your mind when you think about labor and birth.

As you review these positive empowering words, describe the feelings that these words generate (*these empowering words generate the following emotions and sensations within me*).

It is completely natural when thinking about labor to have feelings of both fear and excitement. Wisdom is recognizing that life involves the coexistence of opposites. When a woman surrounds herself with supportive people and creates a safe space around her, she is able to connect with her inner wisdom. By setting aside self-judgment, you can embrace your strength and your vulnerability, your determination and your inclination to surrender.

Stay present to your body and your baby. A conscious birth can be medicated or unmedicated, in a hospital or at home, by cesarean or vaginal birth. It is your powerful, beautiful body that is opening to bring new life into the world. Accept the power that comes from recognizing that your body is an inextricable expression of the universal body. Your mind is a reflection of the cosmic mind. In your willingness to accept the contradictions of birthing a new baby, you gain the opportunity to participate fully in the age-old experience of giving birth to a new life. You are participating in the primordial creative event and will look back on this experience with awe and wonder for the rest of your life.

Exercise

Draw a figure image of yourself as a powerful birthing woman. Show your facial expression and the position you imagine yourself to be in when you birth your baby.

Write the words from your empowering word list many times around the portrait of yourself as a powerful birthing woman. Add whatever additional words you choose from your fearful list, one time each. Hang this picture somewhere in your home where you will see it regularly.

Checklist for a Conscious Birth

Check to see if you are completely comfortable with the following aspects of your birthing experience. If you recognize there is more work required on your part to feel fully prepared, commit to taking the steps to be as ready as possible for your labor and birth.

• I have all the information I need about my birthing site.

• I am aware of and capable of expressing my fears and concerns to my health provider, family, and self.

• I have identified and enrolled my support crew.

• I deeply trust the people who will be supporting me during labor and birth.

• I recognize and accept the fact that there will be times during my labor when I will need to relinquish control of the situation.

• I know it is okay to be noisy during childbirth.

• I know I can work with my body during contractions.

• I know my health care provider will work with me to help create the birth I desire.

• I know I can request pain medications if I need them.

Exercise

Sitting quietly with your eyes closed, center your awareness in the region of your heart. After a few minutes of silence, begin asking yourself the question "What more do I need in order to be fully present and connected to my birthing process?" Continue repeating this question, listening to the messages that emerge from your inner mind. The more innocently you can listen for rather than force a response, the more readily your inner wisdom will make itself known. Take some time to reflect and journal about what you learned.

The Birthing Experience

A woman learns many things about herself during the amazing process of pregnancy and birth. As you reach the end of your pregnancy, approaching labor and birth, envision the process as you would ideally like it to unfold. Seek out the information you need to make fully informed choices.

Imagine yourself standing at the bottom of a mountain with two paths to the top. One path takes you to a chairlift that goes up the mountain, while the other path leads to a hiking trail. Both will get you to the top of the mountain, and each provides you with a unique and memorable experience. The chairlift provides an enjoyable and thrilling ride with little effort or pain. On the chairlift, you will be looking down at the experience and enjoying the scenery. The hike up will be strenuous and challenging, as you are intensely involved with every aspect of the journey. Upon reaching the summit, you will experience a sense of accomplishment.

These are, of course, metaphors for labor. One woman may relish the challenge of giving birth naturally. Another may have no qualms about taking full advantage of modern medical technology. A third woman may be conflicted about the right path for her. The key is to make your choice consciously by using all the information you have gathered, while remaining open to the possibility that sometimes the birthing process takes on a life of its own. There is an Ayurvedic expression that goes "Infinite flexibility is the secret to immortality." We encourage you to have clear intentions for your birth while remaining flexible to all possibilities.

Exercise

Think about your ideal labor. Think about yourself in labor.

Is there a difference between the ideal labor and envisioning yourself in labor? Write a few sentences about what you discover. What more would you need to create your ideal labor?

Moving Through Labor

As you approach the final stages of pregnancy you will naturally have many questions about labor and birth. These are some of the common ones:

How will my contractions feel? Can I handle the pain? How long will I be in labor? Will my partner support me? Will I know how to breathe? Can I trust my body? Will I require medication? Will I need an epidural? Will I have an episiotomy? Will I be able to birth my baby vaginally? Will I need a cesarean? Will my baby be okay?

In this chapter we will explore the process of labor and its many variations to help you prepare for the many possible answers to the many questions in your mind. Let's begin with an overview of the stages of labor.

First Stage of Labor

The onset of progressive mild contractions signals the beginning of the first stage of labor. Each woman experiences these contractions differently. They are mild for some and more intense for others. As the muscles of your uterus contract, the cervix begins to thin (efface) and open (dilate) so your baby can pass through it. During this stage your body will release endorphins to help reduce the sensations of pain as contractions become stronger and closer together.

During *early labor* your cervix will dilate from 0 to 4 centimeters as a result of mild to moderate contractions. These typically last thirty to sixty seconds and may be five to twenty minutes apart. The rest period between contractions varies, lasting from several hours to a day or more.

Perform your normal activities for as long as possible during this period. If it is nighttime, see if you can sleep. You will help your labor to progress by alternating between periods of rest and movement. Trust your instincts to guide you. Relax and follow with your breath. Take walks outdoors or relax in a warm aroma bath if your water has not broken.

As labor progresses into the *active phase*, uterine contractions increase in strength and duration, lasting about sixty seconds and occurring every two to five minutes. During this stage your cervix dilates from 4 to 8 centimeters. As your cervix dilates your baby descends into the pelvic cavity. Contractions become more intense and consume most of your attention. Your awareness shifts inward as your body works harder to open. Endorphins continue to be released throughout your body and your consciousness may slip into an "endorphin haze."

Prepare ahead of time to surround yourself with people who believe in you, so that you are surrounded by safety and love. Breathing, walking, changing positions, making sound, being held, and getting in water will all help you stay as centered as possible.

During the *transition phase* your cervix fully opens as your body prepares to birth your baby. During this phase the sensations in your body become much stronger and more intense. You may feel very vulnerable and doubt that you can go on. The contractions are faster and stronger now as your uterus works to open your cervix from 8 to 10 centimeters. Each contraction may last up to two minutes and occur as frequently as every minute. You may feel you cannot survive the intense experience in one second and then be completely absorbed in it the next. You are at the threshold of bringing your baby into the world.

Second Stage

The second stage begins when the cervix is fully dilated at about 10 centimeters and ends when your baby is born. During this stage your contractions will probably slow down a bit and become less intense, occurring about every three minutes and lasting sixty to ninety seconds. Each contraction helps move your baby down through your birth canal toward your pelvic floor. The urge to push with these contractions may begin before you are fully dilated or it may start five to ten minutes later, although some women never feel a strong urge to push.

CERVICAL DILATION CHART

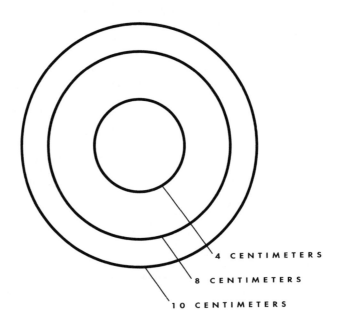

These circles represent
the dilation of the cervix
at four, eight, and ten centimeters.

The sensations of these contractions are powerful. Tiny receptors in the cervical tissues alert your body to release oxytocin in this stage, which facilitates these contractions continuing. The purpose of the contractions shifts from opening your cervix to pushing out your baby. It is common to shift from feelings of exhilaration to exhaustion and back again during this stage. Work with your uterus by bearing down when you feel the urge. Follow the signals from your body and take your time. Have the intention to relax and soften your pelvic floor muscles with each push.

UNDERSTANDING CONTRACTIONS

Each uterine contraction begins at the top of your uterus (fundus), where there is the greatest number of muscle cells. The contraction moves down through the center of your uterus toward your cervix. Throughout labor the upper portion of the uterus is more active and contracts more intensely for a longer period of time than the lower portion of the uterus. The upper uterine segment becomes thicker, while the more passive lower segment becomes thinner.

Contractions are typically mild in early labor and become progressively stronger through active labor and transition. The pain from contractions is due in part to the reduced availability of oxygen to contracted muscle cells, and to the compression of nerves in the lower uterine segment as the cervix is stretched open.

Contractions are the primary power behind the work of labor and birth. You can think of them as waves that start at a lull, build up to a peak, and slowly come back down. They form a regular pattern throughout labor with rest periods in between. The rest periods are important for the laboring woman as well as the unborn baby. Blood flow from the placenta to the womb diminishes with each contraction, but rapidly returns to normal during each rest period. When a woman learns to relax and breathe during rest periods, her baby receives essential nourishment and oxygen.

Exercise

SIMULATING A CONTRACTION

Allow about ten minutes for this exercise. Sit comfortably on the edge of a folded blanket or pillow. Turn on some soothing music and have a clock with a second hand in sight. Now, close your eyes and focus on your breath. Feel the space inside your body and see if you can find your center. Observe your breath entering and leaving your body. Once you have observed your breath for a few cycles, extend your arms out to your sides at about shoulder height with your palms facing down. Begin to flap your arms up and down a few inches about every second or two, keeping your shoulders as soft as you can. Send sound through your body as you breathe out, consciously relaxing the muscles that are not required to perform the exercise. Breathe out through your mouth on your exhalations. Notice what happens to your mind as your arms begin to tire. Keep coming back to your breath and use your sounds. After ninety seconds rest your arms at your sides for about a minute, then repeat the flapping for another ninety seconds. Notice what helps you to relax during the rest periods. Remember to take long, easy breaths to nourish and oxygenate you and your baby. Continue for five to ten cycles, extending and flapping your arms for ninety seconds and then resting for a minute.

CROWNING

Once your baby's head slides under your pubic bone, your perineum will begin to stretch and bulge around your baby's head. This is known as crowning. You may feel a burning sensation, sometimes referred to as "the ring of fire," as a result of the tissues stretching. The burning sensation will subside within a few minutes as the pressure from your baby's head numbs the nerves in your perineum. This feeling is a signal for you to slow down your pushing and begin to ease your baby out slowly. Another push or two and your baby's head will be out of your body. At this point, your baby will turn so that his shoulders can pass under your pubic bone. Your doctor or birthing assistant may help to maneuver your baby's body. Once your baby's shoulders are free, he will slide out of your body and into the world.

PREPARING YOUR PERINEUM

Massaging your perineum with oil weeks before your birth date may help soften the tissues. Use only natural vegetable-based oils, such as sesame, almond, or coconut. During labor, explore different positions that feel comfortable for you and that allow you to stay centered during the final phase of birth. Communicate your needs to your health provider and support team. If it is comfortable, your partner can apply warm cloths with gentle pressure to your perineum during crowning, which may help reduce the chances of your perineal tissues tearing as they stretch. Ask your partner or health care provider to lubricate your perineum with warm oil as your baby is crowning. Push gently to slowly ease your baby out of your body, and if possible, reach down to feel his head so you can stay connected as he emerges from your body.

BIRTHING YOUR BABY

Your body has protected your baby for nine months inside your womb. As he moves through you into the world, do your best to keep him feeling safe, warm, and protected. Have the lights turned down low to give his eyes time to adjust. Keep the room warm so he feels comfortable. Surround him with soft sounds and pleasing aromas. Have him placed immediately on your belly or bring him into your arms so he continues to feel your loving presence. Talk softly to him so that he knows you are there and he is safe. Postpone any necessary invasive procedures for as long as possible.

Third Stage

The surge of emotions you feel holding your newborn baby encourages the release of hormones that stimulate your uterus to contract so you can birth the placenta. Take your time. The umbilical cord and placenta will continue to pulse and bring oxygen to your baby while he is learning to take his first breaths. The cord can be clamped and cut once it has stopped pulsing. After the birth of your baby the placenta begins to slowly separate from your uterine wall. This usually takes about ten to thirty minutes but can sometimes take longer. In a short time your uterus will begin contracting to expel the placenta. The placenta is much smaller than your baby and it usually feels good to push it out of your body.

After You Give Birth

You will have gone through one of the most intense experiences of your life. You will have worked hard for many long hours or even days to bring your baby into the world. You will probably be feeling sweaty, sticky, bloody, exhausted, and ecstatic. Your whole being has been engaged in your baby's birth. Plan ahead to have someone available for you in the first minutes and hours after birth to nurture and protect you. It will take some time for you to recover from the rigors of labor and begin feeling centered again. Your focus shifts from nurturing your baby on the inside to nurturing your baby on the outside. You will need some nutritious food, something replenishing to drink, and a warm washcloth to wipe your face and body.

Strengthening the Bond

In many cultures around the world (and increasingly in the West) babies are placed on their mothers' bellies immediately after birth so Mother and Baby can feel, smell, and touch each other. Parents and babies are meant to be together from birth. Research has shown that important bonding begins within the first minutes and hours after birth, as parents and babies connect with each other through holding, talking, seeing, and touching.

The minutes and hours after birth are magical. Most new parents have difficulty finding the words to describe the depth and intensity of their feelings as they interact with their baby for the first time. As you hold your baby and look into his eyes, you will find yourself falling in love and not wanting to let him go. During the first couple of hours your baby will settle into a "quiet alert state" as he transitions from the womb to the world. He will be awake with his eyes open. After a few hours he will settle into a deep sleep period. Regardless of where you are giving birth, do your best to be with your baby during the first hour or two after birth so you can enjoy these earliest precious experiences with your baby.

Recording Your Experience

If you have the energy during a quiet moment, journal your experiences of labor and birth while they are fresh in your mind. Not only will you enjoy reading these early impressions later on, but years from now your child will have access to your most intimate thoughts and feelings around his arrival. The following is an example of a woman's record of her birthing experience.

The pain of birth is in a completely different category than a broken arm or a toothache. As I journeyed through labor I knew that I was supposed to be feeling these sensations. They were unlike anything I had ever experienced before. I felt like I was working with my body from the first contractions, and as they became stronger, I drifted deeper inside myself. Although I maintained awareness, my mind became completely quiet, and I felt immersed in my own familiar semidarkness.

As I was breathing and moaning, the sounds felt as if they were coming from a deep ancient place inside me. I was on my hands and knees and immersed in warm water. I was able to relax between contractions and let my head hang forward. Sometimes the contractions felt overwhelming and I would moan louder and deeper to release them. I was working hard to stay with the sensations of my body. Opening, breathing, and resting, my body and mind were one. My inner space was my whole reality. I moved and swayed in whatever way felt good.

After a while the contractions got harder and I used my breath and moans to stay with it. As the sensations intensified I started to feel like maybe I couldn't do it. I leaned into the support of my partner and swayed from side to side with my body. My whole being became the contraction.

And then it was time to push. At first little pushes and then all of me was pushing, pushing my baby down through my body. My body was making way. I heard myself moaning. I reached down to feel for my baby's head and there it was, bulging from my body. There was a burning sensation and I breathed into it and then with the next push my baby's head was out, and I was holding and feeling it in my hands. It was so soft and round. My eyes were still closed and I was deep inside feeling everything. I pushed again and my baby came sliding out of me. I opened my eyes and reached down to bring her up into my arms. My eyes closed again. Still deep in the experience I heard my partner say with complete awe and delight, "Oh my God, oh my God! She's here!"

Preparing Yourself

Labor and birth are intense experiences, and having some anxiety as you prepare to birth your baby is completely natural. Acknowledging fears and doubts helps dissipate the power they have over you. Take a few moments now to feel your body and see if you can identify uncomfortable sensations and notice where you are holding apprehension and worry. With your attention on these sensations, use your words to bring to the surface the trepidations you are feeling. Make three lists in your journal, one for the things you are worried about, one for the things you are uncertain about, and one for the things you are doubtful about.

Fear sets into motion the physiology of stress resulting in the release of the powerful chemicals of the fight-or-flight response. Neither the impulse to fight nor the one to run from your contractions serves you well during labor. The hormones of stress constrict the arteries to the uterus and reduce the effectiveness of your contractions. The physiology of fear also has been shown to lower your threshold for pain. Learning to bring yourself from a state of apprehension to one of inner centeredness is a valuable skill that will be of tremendous benefit to you during your birthing experience and throughout your life. Fortunately, you have a precious ally to accomplish this, which is your breath. When you feel out of control, you can come back to your center through conscious breathing.

Using Your Breath

Breathing is the bridge between your mind, body, and baby. As you inhale deeply, you bring nourishment and oxygen into your and your baby's body. As you exhale, you release carbon dioxide and stress. The nourishment of your breath moves deeply into each of your cells and promotes relaxation. Deep, slow breathing can help you release tension from every part of your body. During labor your breath will be your intimate friend, helping you to stay centered, calm, and energized.

These following exercises have been created to bring you a greater awareness of your breath. Become familiar with these simple breathing techniques, which help integrate your mind and body. Choose the exercises that feel right for you and practice them for five to ten minutes per day.

Breathing Exercise #1

ENTRY AND EXIT POINT

As you inhale, imagine your breath as a relaxing mist, calmly coming into your body and filling you with oxygen and nourishment.

As you exhale, imagine your breath releasing slowly down through your body. Feel it helping you to let go of tightness, pain, and tension as it flows out through you. Focus on long, slow exhalations.

Now imagine that you have nostrils somewhere on your belly. Let these imaginary nostrils be your entry and exit point. Close your eyes and rest your hands on your belly. For the next few minutes focus on breathing in and out through your belly nostrils. Allow each in-breath to enter and fill your belly, encircling your baby. As you breathe out, feel your belly muscles soften and allow each out-breath to be long and slow, releasing tension and tightness from your body.

Now imagine your entry and exit point to be your pelvic floor. Closing your eyes, breathe in through your pelvic floor and feel your breath flowing up through your body. Allow it to fill your belly, chest, lungs, and brain with a nourishing mist. As you exhale, allow your breath to gently release and slowly spread down through your body, removing any tension and softening your pelvic floor as it flows out.

Now imagine your entry nostrils to be in a place where you feel most grounded in your body. Let your exit point be through your mouth. As you breathe in, send your breath up through your body toward your throat. As you breathe out, feel the vibration of your breath flowing along your throat and release it with a sigh. Allow your neck and head to hang forward. Soften your shoulders and feel your body becoming loose and limp. Be aware of your chest relaxing and let your belly muscles release.

Try envisioning your entry nostrils at the base of your spine and your exit nostrils at the crown of your head. Bring your breath in through the base of your tailbone and let it slowly flow up along your spine, through the back of your neck, along your head to your crown. As you breath out, send your breath slowly down through your center. Feel it pass through your heart, allowing it to flow around your baby and out your pelvic floor. Focus on long, slow exhalations.

Breathing Exercise #2

ENERGY BREATH

This breath helps bring energy into your body and is beneficial anytime you feel fatigued. It can be helpful throughout the pushing stage of labor and at any other times when you feel tired or need more energy.

As you inhale, imagine your breath to be pure energy entering and filling every cell in your body. Envision each cell tapping from this source the vital energy as your breath expands inside you. As you exhale, allow this energy to flow through you, feeling it revitalize every cell, tissue, and organ in your body.

Breathing Exercise #3

SLOWING DOWN

Close your eyes and take a few minutes to follow and feel your breath as it moves in and out of your body. After a few minutes, have the intention for your breathing to slow down. Do not force any change in your breath. With each inhalation silently repeat the word "slow." With each exhalation, think the word "down." Continue to breathe like this for five to ten minutes, as you mentally repeat the words, "slow down . . . slow down . . . slow down."

As your mind quiets, your body takes over.

Breathing Exercise #4

COUNTING BACKWARD

Close your eyes and focus on your breath. With each succes-
sive inhalation, count backward from 10 to 1. With each
exhalation breath, bring an empowering or affirming word
into your mind. For example, it may go like this:

10 . . . centering

9 . . . relaxing

8 . . . releasing

7 . . . opening

6 . . . accepting

5 . . . surrendering

4 . . . trusting

3 . . . succeeding

2 . . . empowering

1 . . . allowing

Choose the words that work for you. You'll find that this
process quickly brings you back when your mind begins to
race with apprehensions and concerns.

Breathing Exercise #5

HEAD TO TOE

Create a space for yourself with blankets or pillows where you can comfortably lie down. Once you are comfortable, close your eyes and allow your body to begin to relax. Feel your breath moving through you. On your next inhalation bring your breath up through the bottoms of your feet to the top of your head. As you exhale, scan your body from your head to your toes, releasing any tension you may be retaining as you breath out. Repeat this process for five to ten minutes.

Breathing Exercise #6

BREATHING WITH SOUND

Making sounds can help your body relax and open. Moaning, sighing, or groaning with the outflow of your breath creates a soothing vibration that moves through and resonates with your whole body. Find a tone or sound that feels right for you. Many women choose an "ahhh" sound to start. As you exhale, allow your breath to vibrate along your throat and resonate down through your body and out your pelvic floor. Focus on long and slow exhalations. Try sounds that are low pitched and deeply resonant. Continue for five to ten minutes, trying different sounds.

Practice moaning. Let yourself moan. Moaning feels great when you are in labor. There are no fixed rules. There is no one who is going to tell you that you cannot make noise. When contractions get strong, allow yourself to moan and groan. Let it be soft and let it be loud. Close your eyes and go with the sound. Let it feel primitive and let it feel real. Let it be deep and let it feel right. Let it infuse you and let it absorb you. Let it help you open and let it help you soften. Let it help you release and let it help you sink inside. Let it help you move your baby down and let it help you move your baby through.

Staying in Touch

The sense of touch is one of the most important sensory portals to your inner pharmacy. Conscious, nourishing touch can reduce discomfort and calm anxiety. We encourage you to experiment with different touching techniques to learn which ones are most comforting for you.

Your birth partner will be an essential ally to help you stay centered. Explore a variety of styles and pressures with your spouse or partner so you can communicate your needs during labor.

SOFT HANDS

Create a space with blankets and pillows where you can comfortably lie down with your partner sitting beside you. Close your eyes and focus on your breath. After a little while, have your partner gently place his hands over your heart. The touch should be calming and reassuring. As your partner gently lays his hands on you, allow your awareness to receive the love and nurturing that is being sent to you through his hands.

After a few minutes, have your partner move his hands to your belly. As they gently rest on your body, synchronize your breathing together and allow soothing, calming energy to flow from his hands into your body.

Now have your partner place his hands on your head and repeat the process again for several minutes. If there are other places in your body that you would like to be touched, tell your partner to place his hands there. Make a mental note of those places that feel most comforting for you.

Try reversing roles with your partner so you are doing the touching and he is on the receiving end. Touch him in the way that you would like to be touched. Teach your partner how he can be of greatest help to you.

LIGHT TOUCH

Constance Palinsky developed this light-touch technique during her research into pain management and relaxation. It can be used to reduce discomfort in labor and enhance relaxation by invoking pleasure through the surface of the skin. The light-touch technique can also normalize heart rate and blood pressure.

Light touch involves a featherlike massage that may cause goosebumps to arise. Research has shown that this technique enhances the release of oxytocin, the hormone that facilitates labor.

Practice this light-touch massage with your partner during the last month of pregnancy. Notice how it supports deep relaxation and helps you and your partner deepen your connection in preparation for labor.

To practice, lie down with your partner sitting comfortably beside you. After a few moments with your eyes closed, your partner begins stroking the inner surface of your arm from your hand to your underarm. The stroke is very light and is done with either fingernails or fingertips.

After about five minutes, have your partner switch to the other arm. Although the light touch is on the arms, you will find that it has a relaxing effect on your whole body. This technique can also be applied to other parts of the body, including the palms of the hands, the neck and shoulders, and the thighs.

The light-touch technique is very effective when applied to the back. Lie on your side or in Child's Pose leaning over a few pillows. Beginning at your neck, your partner strokes you in a V formation outward from the neck down the back toward the outer edges of the ribs. The strokes continue the entire way down the back to the sacrum. Relax and enjoy the sensations.

Your partner can deepen the calming effect by offering relaxing suggestions as he is lightly stroking you. For example, he might say, "As I stroke your arm, allow your body to soften and relax," or "As you feel each stroke, imagine pain-relieving endorphins releasing and flowing through you."

Lower-Back Counterpressure

As the baby moves deeper into the pelvis during labor, women often experience low-back pressure or deep aching in the lower back. Lower-back discomfort may increase during contractions due to traction on the broad ligaments of the uterus attached to the lower spine. Massage and counterpressure may help to ease this discomfort.

Practice this procedure during the last few weeks of pregnancy so both you and your partner are familiar with the technique and its effects. He can use the heel of his hand, his fist, or a tennis ball.

Lie on your side or rest in Child's Pose with your eyes closed, focusing on your breath.

Tell your partner where you think the pressure would feel the best, which is usually between the lower back and the tailbone. Your partner then presses his hand or tennis ball into your lower back and rotates it in an unhurried circular motion. This is a deep-pressure massage performed slowly with very little movement. Again, switch roles with your partner so he can feel the direct effects and respond to your requests for adjustment. Show your partner how to perform this procedure to provide you with maximum benefit.

STROKING THE SPINE

In this massage, your partner begins by placing the palm of his right hand on your neck along the right side of your spine and slowly slides his hand down your back to your tailbone. He then alternates with his left hand, slowly sliding it down the left side of your spine. This process is repeated several times for about five minutes. Performed with a firm, soothing stroke, this massage can help to ease pain or discomfort during or between contractions.

Creating a Supportive Environment

There are many simple things you can do to make yourself a little more comfortable during your labor. Try some of these suggestions at home, and prepare your "labor support kit" in advance so it will be available to you when you begin having contractions.

AROMA WARM PACK

Warm packs can help relax achy and tense areas in your body. Throughout labor the warmth may be comforting during and in between contractions. Make your own warm pack by filling a clean tube sock with ordinary white rice about three-quarters of the way full. Add half a cup of dried lavender leaves or flowers to the rice, then sew the top of the sock closed. Place the stuffed sock in the microwave for two to three minutes. The sock will remain warm while releasing its aroma scent for about half an hour.

WATER AND JUICE

It is important to stay hydrated while in labor, as dehydration can cause labor to slow down or stall. You will be working hard throughout labor, and it may feel like you are running a marathon. Have plenty of water and fruit juices available. Take a few sips of fluid in between each contraction. Have some liquids with sugar and electrolytes such as Gatorade available to help maintain your energy level, or allow ice chips to melt in your mouth.

FOOD

Eat lightly in early labor so that your body has energy to sustain you throughout birth. If your labor is long and you find that you are hungry, snack on easily digestible foods such as soup, crackers, or frozen fruit ice pops. If you are in a hospital birthing center, be certain to check in with your caregivers and let them know what you feel like eating.

AROMA

Diffuse the aromas that were calming to you throughout pregnancy. The aromas you have associated with relaxation and comfort over the past many months will help calm and soothe you during labor.

DIM LIGHTS

Most mammals seek out dimly lit spaces for the birthing process. A dimly lit room encourages feelings of relaxation and safety. When a woman feels safe and relaxed during labor, oxytocin, the hormone that facilitates contractions, is released and adrenaline, which inhibits contractions, is reduced. A dimly lit room creates an atmosphere conducive to inward focusing.

TUB OR SHOWER

Immersion in warm water can help a laboring woman relax and reduce the level of pain. Similarly, standing or sitting in a warm shower with the rhythmic water spraying on your belly or aching back can help ease your pain so you can flow more easily with your contractions.

MUSIC AND SOUNDS OF NATURE

Listening to soothing music or a recording of sounds from nature can help you relax while in labor. Play music that is soothing and inspiring for you. Try listening to sounds of the ocean, a river, or a waterfall and have tapes and CDs available if they have a calming effect on you.

BIRTHING BALL

Some women find that the use of a large exercise ball about 24 inches in diameter can be helpful during labor. You can purchase one at most health clubs or back stores. Sit on the ball with your feet flat on the floor, and make large circular motions with your hips and pelvis. This movement helps relax the muscles in your back and pelvis. Some women use the ball throughout their entire labor.

Message to Your Birthing Partner

Ask your labor partner to read this next section.

You play an essential role in the birthing process. It is your job to unconditionally support your partner and demonstrate through your words and actions that you believe in her. Stay at your partner's side so she can feel you protecting her birth space. Dim the lights, talk softly, diffuse pleasing aromas, give her water, use warm packs, gently touch her, breathe with her, talk with nurses, handle visitors, and tell her you love her. As labor progresses, continue to look for ways to comfort her.

Have food and drinks available to replenish yourself so that you can stay strong for her throughout the many hours of labor. Draw on other people for support and rest when you need to. Develop a support card so you can continually review opportunities to enhance her comfort level. It may look like the following:

I Will Remind Myself to

- offer her a drink between contractions
- encourage her to empty her bladder

- suggest she try a shower or warm tub bath
- breathe slowly and deeply with her
- make sounds with her
- try using a warm pack
- offer a cold washcloth for her forehead
- walk with her
- suggest touch relaxation
- see if light touch on her arm or back feels good
- apply pressure to her lower back if it is aching
- give her space
- protect her privacy

Birthing Your Way

There is no right or wrong way to birth your baby. As you move into the rigor of contractions, relinquish your attachment to how things should be and simply allow what is unfolding to occur. Be in your body and listen to what it needs. Flow with your breath and slow down. Take one contraction at a time and stay connected with your baby. Feel your support system around you. Listen to your needs, trust your instincts, and release into the process. Release your worries and release your fears. Stay present and trust that your birthing experience is unfolding exactly as it should.

Find Your Birthing Position

Women have different bodies and different needs when it comes to birthing their babies. One position does not fit all. If you move around during labor, you will instinctively find the positions that feel best for you. Although it may not be the norm in your community, upright positions can strengthen uterine contractions and help shorten labor.

We encourage you to try standing, squatting, kneeling, sitting, and getting on your hands and knees. Each of these positions uses gravity to help birth your baby and is worth experimenting with during labor. They may help your baby maneuver his way more easily through your pelvis and birth canal. In between contractions find positions that naturally help you to relax, such as kneeling, leaning forward, Child's Pose, or lying on your side.

STANDING

During early labor you may find you can continue with your normal activities and may benefit from taking a walk. Walking helps your baby descend through your pelvis and encourages efficient contractions. If you are standing while a contraction begins, lean forward and sink into your partner, bed, or the back of a chair. As you bend forward try rocking your pelvis from side to side or move in slow circular motions.

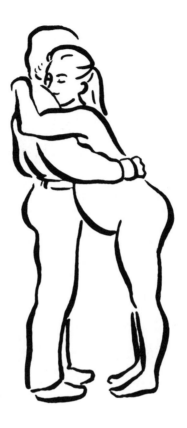

KNEELING

Kneeling can be a useful position throughout labor. Try kneeling with your torso at an upright angle, leaning into your partner. You can also try kneeling and leaning all the way forward into some pillows or blankets. Kneeling is particularly helpful if you are experiencing back labor. While kneeling on your hands and knees, you can easily circle your pelvis or rock it from side to side. This often helps to turn a posterior baby to an anterior position.

SQUATTING

This pose may feel good on and off throughout labor, and can be helpful in speeding up contractions. Some women find squatting to be the most comfortable position and others find that it makes contractions too intense. Squatting encourages the descent of your baby and increases pressure on your cervix. Listen to your body and use this pose only if it feels good. Move out of the squatting position and rest between contractions. Squatting can be helpful during the pushing stage of labor. Making good use of gravity, it creates an effective angle for your baby to descend through your birth canal.

SITTING

Similar to squatting, sitting helps widen your pelvis but usually stimulates less intense contractions. Try sitting facing backward on a chair and lean into the back support. Alternatively, sit at the edge of a chair and relax forward with your arms resting on your thighs. Some women find that sitting on a toilet helps them to relax and soften their pelvic floor muscles.

SIDE LYING

Side lying enables you to be horizontal without having to be on your back. This position can help slow down labor that is going too fast. Place pillows beneath your head, belly, and between your knees for added comfort.

Following your instincts is the most important thing you can do during labor. You may move in and out of many positions during labor, or you might find you primarily use just one. Listen to and trust your body to find the positions that are most effective and comfortable for you.

Affirmations

There may be times during your labor where your thoughts become unconstructive because you are tired, anxious, frustrated, or discouraged. Developing a repertoire of positive affirmations can help you transform negative thoughts into positive ones. Use your affirmations as you exhale, almost like a mantra, to keep your mind focused on thoughts and images that are helpful to your process. These are examples of affirmations that women in labor find useful:

As I release my breath, my cervix softens.
Each contraction is helping me open.
Breathing out, I trust my body.
I inhale strength. I exhale resistance.
Energy comes in. Tension moves out.

Find your own affirmations and write them down. Practice them for a few minutes each day by closing your eyes and thinking of your affirmations as you breathe.

Honoring the Wisdom Within

To accomplish the physiological miracle of labor and birth, your body accesses an inner intelligence that has developed over millions of years of evolutionary time. An essential part of this ancient process is the production and release of natural chemical messengers that facilitate the birthing of your baby. Endorphins and oxytocin are among the most important natural medicines of your inner pharmacy.

ENDORPHINS
Endorphins were discovered as scientists sought to understand why people respond to powerful pain-relieving medications such as codeine or morphine. It was learned that these drugs are effective because they mimic the body's natural pain relievers, known as endorphins. The word *endorphin* is derived from the phrase "endogenous morphine." Endorphins are released when the body needs to alleviate pain, during exercise, during relaxation, and during any activity that generates feelings of comfort, pleasure, or enthusiasm. As a woman progresses through labor, endorphins build in her body to help alleviate discomfort and enhance relaxation. They are more readily released when a woman feels safe and supported.

OXYTOCIN
Oxytocin is a hormone that is produced in the hypothalamus of the brain and released into the bloodstream from the

back portion of the pituitary gland. It is secreted during labor when the fetus stimulates the cervix, causing the uterine muscles to contract. In addition to its effect on the uterus, oxytocin is also important in stimulating the release of milk from your breasts. The most important trigger for the release of oxytocin is physical stimulation of the nipples. There is evidence that oxytocin is also important in mother-baby bonding, as there are brain receptors for oxytocin, which is believed to serve as a facilitating hormone for maternal behavior. Oxytocin is released in short bursts rather than a steady stream and may be inhibited by fear or stress.

When labor is not progressing your doctor may prescribe oxytocin to stimulate your uterus. Stimulating your own nipples may help to increase the strength or frequency of your contractions by naturally enhancing the release of oxytocin.

Honoring Time

In this technological age of nearly instantaneous information, it is easy to forget that natural physiological processes have their own rhythm. Birth has its own clock, and it is important to remember that your baby will be born when your body and baby are ready. Your due date is an approximation, not the final bell at a sporting event. Most people do not birth on their designated day and it is not uncommon to go into labor one to two weeks before or after your due date. Honor the process of your baby coming into the world by allowing your labor and birth to unfold naturally.

The Medical Safety Net

A woman can be connected to her body and baby during birth whether or not she receives medication. The decision to receive medical intervention does not imply that you become a passive participant in your birthing experience. Even if you require medicines during labor and delivery, you can be powerfully present as you birth your baby.

Human beings have been birthing babies for hundreds and thousands of years. With the advent of modern obstetrical care, there has been an increased tendency to intervene sooner, which may not always be in the best interest of Mother and Baby. The safety net provided by modern medicine is invaluable; and yet, a worthy goal is to reduce the need for medical intervention.

Education and preparation enable women to have expanded choices in the birth process, allowing them to make informed decisions for themselves and their babies. It is helpful that you understand the possible challenges that may arise during labor so that you can be an active participant in your own care. If labor fails to progress, if the pain becomes unbearable, if exhaustion takes over, or if there are signs that the baby is in distress, the medical safety net is there for you. Let's review the most common medical interventions that may arise during the birthing process.

External Fetal Monitoring

External fetal monitoring is routinely used in most hospitals to keep track of fetal heart rate and uterine contractions. A monitor may be strapped around your belly for twenty minutes of every hour in a hospital setting. During normal contractions there is a temporary decline in oxygen delivery to the baby, resulting in a slight drop in your baby's heart rate, which returns to normal during rest periods. The monitor records these patterns for your care provider with the goal of reducing the risk of problems with the baby, while maintaining the lowest possible rate of medical intervention.

Unfortunately, there are studies showing that close monitoring leads to increased rates of cesarean deliveries, which is not always beneficial to Mother or Baby. If your labor is monitored, play an active role in the decision-making process. If monitoring shows that your baby is in distress, try potentially helpful measures such as changing your position, turning from side to side, receiving supplemental oxygen, and, if you are receiving Pitocin, asking for it to be turned off. Clearly, if these simple measures do not relieve the problem, be open to whatever is necessary to have the best outcome for you and your baby.

Intravenous Access

Intravenous (IV) access through a catheter is considered routine at many hospitals in order to keep the laboring mother hydrated and to provide access for other fluids and medication should the need arise. If you are birthing in a hospital setting, discuss the IV policy with your health care provider. There are studies showing that women who are well hydrated have faster labors than those who are not. If it is an option, see if you can maintain the necessary hydration by drinking water and juices during labor. An IV can always be started if at some point you need to receive medications. Our experience is that mothers empowered to trust the wisdom of their birthing bodies will drink adequate fluids throughout labor, particularly if their partners remind them.

Pitocin to Induce or Augment Labor

To assist in the stimulation of contractions or to advance labor that is slow to progress, Pitocin, a synthetic form of the pituitary hormone oxytocin, may be given intravenously. Your body naturally produces oxytocin in short bursts during labor to facilitate contractions, but Pitocin is administered intravenously in a continuous flow. As a consequence, it may produce unusually strong contractions. Continuous monitoring is required with Pitocin to be certain that the strong contractions are not restricting blood flow to the baby. Due to the strength of the Pitocin-induced contractions, women who receive it more commonly require stronger pain medications, including epidural anesthesia.

There are clearly times when Pitocin is required to stimulate labor, and its appropriate use may reduce the need for a cesarean delivery. On the other hand, it is not a drug that should be used casually. It is difficult to support the increasingly commonplace choice to induce labor with Pitocin merely for convenience' sake. Electively induced labors are associated with a higher incidence of cesarean deliveries, forceps deliveries, and epidural anesthesia. Become informed about the benefits and the risks before you allow a drug to be administered to your body.

Natural Alternatives to Stimulate Labor

If labor progress is slow, it's worth trying to enhance your contractions with natural approaches before proceeding with Pitocin. Check with your care provider before using these techniques to stimulate your labor.

ACUPUNCTURE AND ACUPRESSURE

A number of reports have suggested that acupuncture, acupuncture electrostimulation, and acupressure may stimulate labor if your cervix has begun to soften and thin. Although the science is still in its infancy, there is no risk to stimulating a few acupuncture points. Two points have been

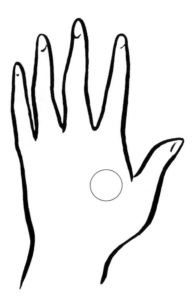

reported to enhance labor, one on the hands and another above the ankles. *Large Intestines 4 (Ho-Ku)* is located on the back of the hand in the muscular web between the thumb and index finger; *Spleen 6 (San-Yin-Chiao)* is on the inner surface of the lower leg, about 3 inches above the major protruding bone on the inner surface of the ankle.

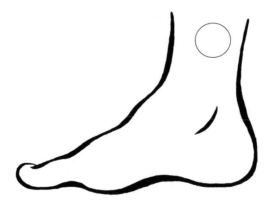

Have your partner stimulate these points by firmly massaging them with his thumb for a minute at a time. The pressure should verge on feeling uncomfortable. He should alternate stimulating the points on your upper and lower extremities on both the left and right sides.

MAKING LOVE

It has been said, "What got the baby in can help get the baby out." Oxytocin is released during a woman's orgasm, and prostaglandins are contained in a man's semen. Both of these chemicals help stimulate contractions and soften the cervix. Do not have sex if your water has broken.

NIPPLE STIMULATION

Nipple stimulation results in the release of the hormone oxytocin from your pituitary gland, which facilitates contractions to begin or continue. Lightly caress your nipples or have your partner lick or suck on them. You want to be careful not to overstimulate your uterus, so begin by stimulating only one nipple at a time for a few minutes every few hours.

Prostaglandin Gel

A gel made up of a synthetic prostaglandin has been shown to ripen the cervix and induce labor when applied to the vagina. In a number of studies, women receiving this prostaglandin gel called *misoprostol* had less need for epidural analgesia, Pitocin stimulation, and cesarean delivery. It can cause uterine stimulation. If you are considering inducing your labor, discuss the possibility of using this prostaglandin gel as an option.

Epidural Analgesia

The epidural space is a little gap between the bones of your spine and the sack that holds the spinal cord and nerves. Pain-relieving medication is administered into the epidural space through a thin plastic catheter, placed by an anesthesiologist through a needle. The needle is removed and the catheter is left in place. The tubing is connected to a pump, which continuously infuses the medication. When anesthetic medication is dripped around the spinal nerves, pain signals from the body are blunted.

A woman usually begins feeling numb within five to ten minutes after the medication is infused. An intravenous line is required and her mobility is limited. Because epidural analgesia may slow labor, Pitocin is more commonly required. Although epidural analgesia is routine in many birthing centers and there is a trend toward lower doses of medicine, this procedure is associated with longer labors and a greater chance of requiring instruments during the birth. In large studies, babies born to women receiving epidural analgesia have lower Apgar scores, a measurement of newborn health. However, babies whose mothers received epidural analgesia generally are healthier at birth than those whose mothers received narcotic medications.

There is not a clear right or wrong answer to the question of epidural analgesia. For many women, the pain relief is worth the small increased risks. Others choose to handle the pain of labor through natural means. We encourage you to inform yourself of the pros and cons of epidural analgesia, so you can make a conscious choice for yourself and your baby.

Narcotics

A narcotic will take the edge off your pain, although it will seldom eliminate it altogether. These strong pain-relieving medicines are given either intravenously or into a muscle. Intravenous medication takes effect faster but does not last as long as intramuscularly administered narcotic medications. It is common to feel drowsy and queasy for a while after receiving narcotics.

Narcotic medications enter your baby's bloodstream soon after you receive them and, at high levels, can affect your baby's blood pressure and breathing. If there are residues of narcotic medications in your baby's body at birth, he may have a weak sucking response for a few days. Try using the least amount of narcotic drugs necessary to provide adequate pain control, and try limiting narcotics as you get closer to birthing your baby.

Episiotomy

An episiotomy is a ½- to 1-inch incision made in the perineum during crowning to enlarge the opening through which your baby passes. The incidence of this surgical procedure varies widely. In some birthing centers episiotomies are performed in as few as 20 percent of births, whereas in other units the procedure is used in more than 70 percent of births. Although overall rates have been dropping over the past twenty years, a report from Thomas Jefferson University in Philadelphia suggested that this procedure should be required in less than one in five vaginal births. Rather than reducing the chance for more serious tears, most surveys have actually suggested a higher risk in women undergoing episiotomies.

Studies have suggested that the position of a woman at the time of birth correlates with the risk of perineal tearing. The most important issue is that a woman listens to her body and finds the position that feels right to her. Rather than accepting the view that one position fits all, we encourage you to move around until you find the best one for you. In some studies, giving birth in a side position had the lowest risk of injury.

Well in advance of your birth, have a conversation with your health care provider about his or her usual practice regarding routine episiotomies and your personal preferences. When women are encouraged to push at their own pace and assume a pushing position that feels comfortable for them, the incidence of tearing or requiring an episiotomy is reduced. A recent report from Australia found that the episiotomy rate among obstetricians was five times higher than the rate among midwives, suggesting that allowing labor to unfold at its own pace can reduce the need for medical intervention.

Cesarean Birth

Cesarean section (c-section) is the surgical delivery of a baby through an incision in a woman's abdomen and uterus. Almost one in four babies in America are born through cesarean section, although it is generally accepted that in low-risk pregnancies, the rate should be closer to one in seven. The term *cesarean* comes from the belief that Julius Caesar was born that way.

If, for a number of reasons, a baby cannot safely be birthed vaginally, cesarean delivery may be indicated. If the baby's head is too large, the placenta is blocking the cervix, or labor fails to progress, for example, a c-section may be the best option. Cesarean birth rates vary widely across the world, highlighting the different thresholds for resorting to a surgical delivery. Although in the past it was believed that "once a cesarean, always a cesarean," there is now good evidence that 60 percent to 80 percent of women who previously delivered by c-section are capable of a safe subsequent vaginal birth. There are many advantages to going the vaginal route, including shorter hospital stays, faster recovery, lower infection risk, and less need for blood transfusions.

If despite your best intentions and efforts, it is determined that a c-section is necessary, the procedure will take place using either spinal or epidural anesthesia, and you will be awake for your baby's birth. If the cesarean is an emergency, you may be given general anesthesia to put you to sleep. A nurse will shave your abdominal and upper pubic area, and an IV will be started in your arm to give you fluids and necessary medications. You will also have a urinary catheter inserted to keep your bladder empty.

Once you have received this initial preparation, you will be taken into the delivery room where your abdomen will be washed with antiseptic solution and covered with sterile drapes. The surgeon will then make an incision in your abdomen. You might feel some pressure and hear some unfamiliar sounds as this is done, but should not feel any pain. Your baby will then be lifted out of your body and into the world. The time from incision to the birth of your baby is usually about ten minutes. Repair of your incision will take another thirty to forty-five minutes.

Ask your doctor if the drapes can be lowered so you can see your baby coming into the world. Upon arrival your baby's mouth and nose will be suctioned and then he will be brought over to a warming table to be checked. Your partner can be right there with him. After these initial procedures, your baby will be snuggled up in a blanket and brought to you for a few minutes. While your placenta is being removed and your wound is being closed, your baby may be brought to a warming bed or another room for additional observation. Your partner can stay with your baby during these procedures. Once your surgery is completed, you will be brought to another room where you will recover.

Consider the possibility of having a cesarean delivery and think about how you can make this experience as positive as possible. You are not just having surgery; you are giving birth to your baby. If you are having an elective cesarean, create a special ritual for the morning of your baby's birth. Place candles around you and your partner, connecting with each other and your baby on this day of his birth. Read a poem or say a few words to invite your baby into the world. Sleep with one of his baby blankets against your body the night before your cesarean so that it smells like you on the morning of his arrival. Bring this blanket with you to the hospital and have him snuggled in it once he is born. See if your partner can take pictures and ask for your baby to be brought to you as soon as possible.

The most important aspect of your recovery from a c-section is having people to support you. Surround yourself at the hospital and home with people who can mother you. Most women stay in the hospital for two to four days and require several weeks to fully recover from the surgery. Your baby will be looking for his connection to you, listening for your voice, and seeking the comfort of your familiar smell. Keep him close by as you recuperate.

The Amazing Story of Birth

Birth is a time of power and surrender, of beginnings and endings, of primordial feelings and absolute novelty. Your personal birth story echoes the stories of women since the beginning of humankind, yet it can be entirely unique. Allow yourself to be present for the most amazing experience of your life. Here is one woman's story:

After hours of early labor, my contractions escalate. As they continue to build, the waves of sensations become stronger and there are only a few minutes' rest period between each one. I begin thinking to myself, "This is really hard, maybe I can't do this."

As I breathe through another contraction, I feel my body leaning into my partner's. I look up into his eyes and I see that he is here with me, and I think to myself, "I can do this."

I change positions, following my breath as I settle back inside. I listen to my body, and as I feel myself breathing, I let go into the sensations. As the pain intensifies, doubt comes up again and I think, "This is much harder than I remember . . . I can't do it."

My partner holds me in his arms and I hear my health provider say, "I know it's hard, but you're doing great. Everything is fine and your body is working perfectly."

I go back inside my body, feeling each contraction taking me beyond the boundary where I thought I couldn't go. I'm moaning and breathing as my body opens. I begin to cry and I let myself lose control as I groan. I think, "I don't know how much longer I can keep this up."

The sensations are overwhelming. I feel like I want to throw up and my lower back is aching. My partner presses his hand into my back to help ease the pain and I feel the first urge to push. I soften my body and begin bearing down. The sensations are powerful and the urge is strong. With each push I feel my baby moving deeper.

After a while, my health provider tenderly strokes my hair and says, "Little pushes now. Your baby's head is right here. Reach down and feel her. Just a few more pushes and she will be here."

And I can feel my baby's head at the threshold of birth. Another push and she comes through me into the world. I cuddle her to my chest and hold her in my arms for the first time. As I look into her eyes, I think, "This is the most amazing thing I have ever done. I gave birth to this beautiful baby!"

Enliven Through Your Attention

• Place your hands on your belly a few times throughout the day and send loving thoughts to your unborn baby.

• Journal each day about your experiences.

• Early in your pregnancy, plant a tree or flowering bush to symbolize the growth of your baby in the womb. After your child is born, you can take care of the plant together.

• Read enchanting stories and heartfelt poetry aloud to your baby and listen to beautiful, relaxing music each day.

• Perform a daily oil massage on yourself before you bathe or shower.

• Diffuse an aroma while listening to music, while soaking in a tub, or while meditating to create the association between the fragrance and the relaxed state of awareness.

• Ensure that you have all six tastes available during your meals throughout the day.

• Choose to eat meals that are rich in color, aroma, and texture.

• Be mindful as you eat your meals. Eat at least one meal each week in silence with your full awareness.

• Practice meditation for twenty to thirty minutes twice daily.

• Pay attention to signals of stress that you experience during the day and employ stress-reducing behaviors to minimize the harmful effects of stress on you and your unborn baby.

• Perform yoga postures with awareness on a regular basis, being gentle and respectful of your body.

• Embrace your pregnancy as an opportunity to experience more natural healing approaches to common minor health concerns.

• Whenever an uncomfortable symptom arises, go through a mental checklist to ensure that you are taking time to relax, eating properly, drinking enough fluids, and exercising regularly.

• Develop an open line of communication with your health care provider and have a low threshold for calling about any emotional or physical concern that may arise.

• Commit to improving your conscious communication skills. When you are feeling upset, determine what you really need and ask for the behavior that will fulfill your need.

• Practice the seven steps for emotional clearing when you are experiencing emotional turbulence. Notice how empowering the process can be when you take responsibility for your feelings.

• Whenever you are finding it difficult to communicate with your partner about your feelings, create the opportunity to practice conscious listening.

• Become familiar with the stages and phases of labor and birth. Knowing the map will increase the likelihood that you get to where you want to go.

• Practice your breathing exercises so you can draw upon a wide range of centering techniques during labor.

• Explore with your birthing partner various massage, pressure, and breathing practices so you can build confidence that he will be there for you when you need his assistance.

CHAPTER 8

Nurturing Mother and Baby

Ever present, all pervading

All knowing, eternal, causeless.

Grander than the grandest,

Smaller than the small.

You begin your journey as a speck of intelligence.

Food, images, memories, and desires

Transform you into cells, eyes, ears, and flesh.

Curving back within yourself,

You create again and again.

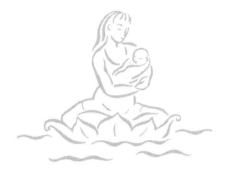

You are the lover and the beloved,

The seer and the scenery,

The creator and the creation.

Behold this child from the womb of creation.

Through the seed of man,

To the womb of woman,

You return to us again and again,

Ever dancing your cosmic dance.

—DEEPAK CHOPRA

our baby's birth is a magical beginning. You have been the chief participant in a creative process through which a new life has become manifest. The next days, months, and years will be devoted to nurturing your baby so that she can realize the full potential of being human.

Incubating and birthing a baby may be the most amazing and intense experience of your life. Following pregnancy and birth it is common to feel a combination of bliss and exhaustion. Please take the time to consciously slow down and honor yourself, your partner, and your baby. Create the space over the next few weeks to relax, meditate, and sleep as much as you can, allowing your rhythms and those of your newborn to entrain. The more you rest, the more you will be able to enjoy your new baby. To accomplish this, you'll need to temporarily relinquish your need to keep everything else in life under control, making bonding with your baby and rejuvenating yourself your highest priorities.

Give yourself permission to let go of cleaning and household errands for a while. The first few postpartum weeks go by incredibly fast. Slow down and enjoy each moment. Create a peaceful sanctuary around you and your baby. Take time to close your eyes and breathe. Try not to rush off to the next stage before you fully experience the one you're in. Surround yourself with relaxing music and soothing aromas. Set up a support system to help with meals, cleaning, and errands so that you can focus your energy on caring for your baby and for yourself. Your body needs time to adjust to the dramatic physiological changes that occur after birth. Honor your body by giving it time to heal.

Strengthening the Bond

Parents and newborn babies are meant to be together. The intimacy between a mother and baby during the nine months inside the womb needs to continue outside the womb through feeding, cuddling, rocking, holding, and carrying. Babies have a primordial need to feel physically connected to their caregivers and seek this intimate bond soon after birth. Fathers and partners can share in this intimacy from the first minutes of life.

In most cultures across time and throughout the world, Baby, Mother, and Father are nurtured and pampered during the immediate postpartum period. The nuclear family is surrounded with protection and support by their extended family and community. Friends and family members bring nutritious meals and perform basic household chores, enabling the new parents to get some rest so they can be emotionally available to bond with their new baby. One of the challenges of modern Western society is overcoming the isolation that our uprooted lifestyle can engender. Well in advance of your baby's birth make preparations for family and friends to be available to support you during the first few weeks after birth. According to Ayurveda, the first six weeks after giving birth is a critical period for the mother. Taking time to replenish yourself after the powerful expenditure of energy during pregnancy and birth prevents imbalances from setting in that can lead to health concerns later in life.

Immediately After Birth

Think *rejuvenation* and *replenishment* after birth. Be sure to drink plenty of fresh juice, water, or herbal tea to hydrate yourself. Listen to your appetite and when it kicks in, begin with easily digestible soups or hot cereals, advancing to more substantial foods as you feel hungrier. Ask your support team to prepare delicious, nutritious, freshly prepared meals when you are ready. Spend a few minutes several times per day gently massaging your belly with warm oil. Almond, sesame, coconut, and jojoba oils are good choices. Take as much rest as possible with your baby and partner. For the first several days at the hospital, birthing center, or home, sleep when your baby sleeps. Stay in your pajamas day and night for the first week. Although you will be tempted to use your baby's downtime to catch up on things, we encourage you to make getting the rest you need a high priority. Spend a few minutes tape-recording or journaling your impressions about the birth experience while the thoughts and feelings are fresh in your mind. Continue this ritual of documenting the process, which you will thoroughly enjoy reading months and years from now.

The First Few Weeks

After the intensity of the labor and the first few days following birth, you will probably be looking forward to quiet time with your baby. Focus on recovering your energy by staying close to home for the first few weeks. Have someone available to nurture and support you so you can concentrate your attention on your baby. Again, make resting a high priority.

Meditate as much as you can. If you are up during the night feeding your newborn, practice your breathing-awareness meditation so your body is resting even if your mind is awake. Cultivate the habit of giving yourself and your baby a daily warm oil massage, focusing extra attention on your belly and head. For the first few weeks, be gentle with your digestive tract. Favor simple, nourishing foods like soups, steamed vegetables, casseroles, and freshly baked breads. Be sure to continue drinking plenty of fluids including fresh juices and warm herbal teas, particularly if you are breastfeeding. Continue paying attention to the sounds, sights, and smells in your environment, choosing to expose you and your baby to sensory impulses that are nourishing while avoiding those that are toxic.

Comfort for Your Perineum

Expect to experience some soreness in your perineum after a vaginal birth. To soothe the tissues that have been traumatized from abrasions, stitches, tears, or bruising, use frozen herbal pads on your perineum to reduce swelling and discomfort. *To make the herbal ice packs, steep one or more of the herbs mentioned below for five to ten minutes in hot water. Strain the herbal mix and place it in a container. When it is cool, add a few capfuls of liquid aloe vera. Soak large sanitary pads in the herbal mix, seal the soaked pads in separate plastic bags, and freeze*. We recommend that you make these up a few weeks before your due date and store them in your freezer.

There are a number of different herbs that can be effective in relieving perineal discomfort. Try boiling 1 teaspoon of fresh grated ginger (*Zingiber officinale*) in a pint of water, soaking a sanitary pad in the decoction, sealing it in a plastic bag, and chilling the pad before extracting it from the bag and applying it to the perineal region. German chamomile (*Matricaria recutita*) has a soothing effect on irritated tissue. Make an infusion using 1 tablespoon of flowers per cup of boiling water. Cool and apply compresses with a clean cotton cloth or pad. Witch hazel (*Hamamelis virginiana*) is derived from a bush that is native to the forests of Atlantic North America. It is commonly helpful in reducing symptoms of minor skin irritations and inflammations. There are a number of commercial witch hazel preparations available through your local pharmacy. You can make up your own by pouring a cup of boiling water over a couple of tablespoons of dried leaves, then straining after ten minutes. Apply soothing compresses after the infusion is cool. Witch hazel is also helpful to relieve swollen hemorrhoids.

Use a squirt bottle filled with warm water and a few drops of Betadine solution to ease discomfort and keep your perineum clean. Squirt the warm water solution over your perineum each time after you urinate. Aloe vera gel can be helpful to relieve perineal soreness. Apply the inner gel from a fresh leaf or prepared aloe vera gel directly to any irritated area. It can help relieve pain and protect the healing area from infection.

Bleeding

After your baby is born, you will have a bloody discharge called lochia, which usually lasts for about six weeks. During the first week the flow will be similar to your menstrual period, and then it should gradually lighten over the next few weeks. Your uterus will take about six to eight weeks to return to its normal size while the site where the placenta was attached heals. Take it easy throughout these first few weeks to help your body heal. Use sanitary napkins rather than tampons during this time.

Afterbirth Contractions

For one or two days after birth you may experience contractions as your uterus slowly returns to its normal size. Women who have had prior pregnancies may more commonly experience these as their wombs need to work a little harder to get back into shape. These contractions are commonly felt during breastfeeding, because the natural hormone oxytocin that stimulates your milk letdown also helps to contract your uterus. If these sensations become uncomfortably intense, try practicing the following exercise.

Exercise

As you feel a contraction, close your eyes and take in a long, slow breath. With each exhalation visualize your body relaxing from your head down into your toes. After a few breaths bring your awareness to your belly. Feel your belly rise and fall around your womb. With your next breath allow your awareness to drift inside your womb. Sense your breath flowing through this sacred space inside of you—this place from which your baby has just come. Acknowledge your womb for all its work and wisdom in nourishing and birthing your baby. Honor it now for continuing to work as it returns to its normal size.

There are a couple of herbs that may be helpful in relieving the discomfort of postpartum contractions.

• Raspberry *(Rubus idaeus)* has a long traditional use in soothing and balancing the female reproductive tract. A tablespoon of the leaves steeped in a cup of hot water can help relieve cramping and soothe the digestive system.

• Valerian root *(Valeriana officinalis)* has been used since the Middle Ages to relieve discomfort and reduce tension. It has been shown to relieve muscle spasms and can be sedating. Because it may enter into breast milk, it should be used sparingly in breastfeeding moms. It can be added to a hot bath soak to relieve muscle aches.

Hemorrhoids

Hemorrhoids are common after giving birth. These swollen rectal veins can be quite uncomfortable and bothersome. They frequently develop during pregnancy due to the excess weight of the womb on your pelvic floor. The pressure from the intense pushing during labor can often make them worse. Although they usually disappear within a few weeks after birth, they can sometimes persist longer. Do your best to avoid straining during bowel movements, using a gentle stool softener if you are constipated. Be certain to get enough fiber in your diet through plenty of fresh fruits, vegetables, and whole grains. The following suggestions can also help reduce discomfort and swelling.

• Aloe vera gel can be applied directly to the hemorrhoids to help reduce swelling and soothe discomfort. Use the gel from a freshly cut leaf or a packaged product from your health food store or pharmacy.

• Psyllium seeds (*Plantago afra*) have been used throughout Asia, Europe, and the Mediterranean since antiquity to support smooth bowel movements. They are very mucilaginous and swell to ten times their size when fluids are available. Metamucil is the most common commercial form of psyllium. It is important to drink plenty of fluids when taking psyllium.

• Licorice root (*Glycyrrhiza glabra*) can be useful in the short-term treatment of hemorrhoids. Licorice has antiinflammatory properties and has been used traditionally to soothe the digestive tract. Taken in excess, it can lead to elevated blood pressure and altered blood electrolytes. A cup of tea made from 1 teaspoon of shredded root per day for a couple of weeks will provide a safe dose.

• Witch hazel pads already packaged or made by soaking gauze pads in a witch hazel solution can provide hemorrhoid comfort. Chill the pads in the refrigerator and apply to your bottom after a bowel movement or as needed for comfort.

• Take a warm sitz bath in which you immerse only your legs, buttocks, hips, and lower abdomen in warm water. The name comes from the German word *sitzen* meaning "to sit." A variety of soothing herbs can be added to the bathwater, including calendula (marigold), lavender, rosemary, chamomile, marshmallow, and slippery elm. Aveena oatmeal, available in most pharmacies, can also be added to a bath. Add about 1 cup of herbs to the warm bathwater and soak for fifteen to twenty minutes.

Pelvic Floor Exercises—Kegels

Developed by Dr. Arnold Kegel in the 1940s, these pelvic floor exercises will help you strengthen and regain tone in the muscles of your perineum. They can aid in the recovery of trauma from stitches or tears. At first you may find it hard to hold these muscles for more than a few seconds, but continue performing fifty to one hundred Kegel exercises each day, and over a few weeks you will find that your perineal muscles regain their normal strength. When toned, these muscles help support your internal organs and prevent urine incontinence now and throughout your life. (See Chapter 4, page 122, for instructions on performing Kegels.)

The Emotions of Motherhood

Your emotions may fluctuate widely during the first few weeks after your baby's birth. One minute you may feel indescribably happy as you look into the eyes of your baby and in the next minute you may feel overwhelmed with sadness. You may find yourself crying and laughing in the same breath without knowing why. Rapid changes in moods are a normal feature of the postpartum period. This emotional turbulence is generated by the many biochemical and hormonal changes that occur in your body after birth.

As your mind quiets, your body takes over.

The fatigue that commonly accumulates as a result of your baby's irregular sleep schedule is an important contributing factor. This typical phase of uncomfortable emotional turbulence commonly known as the "baby blues" usually subsides within ten days to two weeks of birth. The following suggestions can help you settle these emotional waves.

• Get as much rest as possible. Sleep when Baby sleeps or nap when older children nap.

- Meditate daily—you can do this while feeding your baby.
- Don't skip meals—eat fresh, nourishing foods daily.
- Begin exercising as soon as it is safe. Start with leisurely strolls, gradually increasing your level of activity.
- Accept loving support from your family and friends.
- Communicate your concerns to your spouse or partner, to close friends, and to your health advisor.
- Journal your thoughts and feelings on a daily basis.

Depression

Although as many as 80 percent of women have a short bout of the baby blues after delivering their child, postpartum depression is a more serious concern. Affecting about 10 percent of new mothers, it is more severe and intense and may affect the ability to care for a baby. Women with a prior history of depression are more susceptible, but it can affect any woman, regardless of age or number of prior pregnancies.

Postpartum depression may not become obvious until several days or weeks after birth. A woman may find herself overwhelmed with sadness, irritability, and exhaustion to the point that she is unable to perform basic household chores or function productively at work. She may lose the ability to enjoy things that used to bring her pleasure and may be overcome with feelings of anxiety. Sleep and eating patterns are often disrupted. In extreme cases, a woman may have impulses to harm herself or her newborn baby. Her embarrassment over her feelings adds insult to injury and may delay her seeking necessary treatment.

Lack of social support along with an unrealistic need to be a perfect mother increases the risk for postpartum depression. Complications during pregnancy and a premature birth may also be contributing factors.

The most important thing to recognize if you are having intense feelings of sadness is that you need and deserve professional help. If you know someone who is suffering with this condition, strongly encourage her to get the attention she needs. The most loving and caring individuals may find themselves struggling with depression. If you are having this problem, it does not mean that you are a bad person; it does not mean that you do not love your baby; it does not mean that you are being punished for something you did or did not do. It *does* mean that you have a physiological and biochemical imbalance that needs treatment. For your sake and the sake of your baby, get the support you need to overcome this distressing condition if you find yourself experiencing the following symptoms for longer than two weeks after giving birth to your baby:

- persistent feelings of exhaustion
- increasing feelings of sadness, guilt, or helplessness
- lack of interest in your baby
- inability to care for yourself
- intense feelings of anger with thoughts of harming yourself or your baby

Help with postpartum depression can take the form of counseling and, if appropriate, antidepressant medication. As your spirits begin to lift, good lifestyle practices can help you reawaken your inner pharmacy so you can regain your sense of self and enjoy the experience of mothering your baby.

Breastfeeding

Your milk is specifically made for your baby. It is far superior to any other fluid that you could use to feed her. Breast milk is a remarkable fluid, infused with the best nutrients for your baby's well-being. In addition to supplying core nutritional needs of your baby, breast milk has components that provide immune protection against a wide range of illnesses and infections. It enhances the development of healthy bacteria in your baby's digestive tract and reduces her risk for allergies and asthma as your child develops. Although the digestive enzymes in your baby's stomach break down some of the substances in breast milk, others provide a level of protection that cannot be replicated by formula.

The first few days after your baby is born, your breasts produce colostrum. This is a yellow-colored, concentrated fluid, rich with infection-fighting antibodies. These antibodies attach to the lining of your baby's nose, mouth, throat, and stomach, protecting her from various viruses and bacteria. Enzymes to improve digestion, growth factors to support healthy gut bacteria, and proteins that regulate iron are all contained in colostrum. It also has a mild laxative quality, which helps your baby move the first stools of meconium out of her body. By the third or fourth day after birth, your breasts will begin the shift from producing colostrum to producing mature milk. The milk produced during this shift is known as transitional milk. The concentration of immunoglobulins and total protein decreases during this transition while the lactose, fat, and calorie content increases. This transformation takes place over a period of about two weeks.

The composition of mature milk changes throughout each feeding. The milk at the start of a feeding is called foremilk, which is high in volume but low in fat content. The milk toward the end of a feeding is called hindmilk. It is

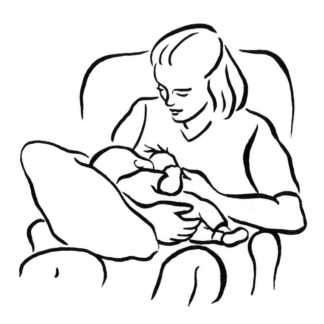

higher in fat content but lower in volume. Breast milk provides high levels of long-chain fatty acids, which are important in healthy brain development, and carnitine, which is important in energy metabolism. Allowing your baby to feed for as long as she likes ensures that she receives both the necessary volume and the fat content for healthy development.

Herbs to Enhance Milk Supply

Although it is generally recognized that infants benefit from being fed breast milk for at least the first year of life, many woman discontinue breastfeeding sooner. A reason commonly cited for stopping breastfeeding is the mother's concern that she is not producing enough milk to satisfy her baby's needs. Although scientific validation is mostly lacking, there are a number of herbs traditionally suggested to enhance a mother's milk production.

- Fenugreek (*Trigonella foenum-graecum*) is the most commonly recommended milk-boosting herb. It is available in the form of tablets, tinctures, and teas. It does have a documented blood sugar–lowering effect, so be certain to eat regularly throughout the day if you are trying fenugreek. In high doses, fenugreek can give your breast milk (and your baby) the smell of maple syrup.
- Aromatic herbs such as fennel (*Foeniculum vulgare*), anise (*Pimpinella anisum*), and cinnamon (*Cinnamomum verum*) each

have their proponents as milk-enhancing herbs. Perhaps they add interesting flavors and fragrances to the milk, resulting in more vigorous suckling and enhanced milk production. They also have digestive calming effects, which can be of benefit to both Mother and Baby.

• Alfalfa (*Medicago sativa*) is an herb traditionally used for rejuvenation that also is reputed to enhance milk supply. It is naturally rich in vitamins A, D, E, and K.

• The Ayurvedic herb Shatavari (*Asparagus racemosus*) is a cousin to the common asparagus plant. Shatavari has a long-standing reputation as a rejuvenative for women and as a breast milk enhancer, with studies in cattle documenting its milk-augmenting properties. Eat your asparagus and see if your supply increases.

Flowing with Nourishment

According to Ayurveda, breast milk is an *upadhatu*, or "superior byproduct," of a woman's *rasa*, which can be translated as plasma, sap, or essence. In order for breast milk to be nourishing, a woman's *rasa* must be appropriately nourished. The best way to ensure that your "sap" is nourished is to be certain that you are eating a well-rounded balanced diet with appropriate levels of protein, carbohydrates, fats, vitamins, minerals, and fiber. Listening to your appetite and following a balanced six-taste diet is the easiest way to confidently receive the nourishment you need from the food you are eating. We also recommend you continue with a high-potency multivitamin/multimineral to provide a nutritional safety net as long as you are breastfeeding. Be sure to drink plenty of fresh water and juices while avoiding nutritionally empty sodas, coffee, and alcohol.

Feeling comfortable with and confident about breastfeeding supports adequate milk production. Taking time to meditate (it's great to do so while breastfeeding), finding a quiet space, and visualizing your nourishment flowing easily from you to your baby can all help you relax into the experience. Seek guidance from a lactation counselor if you are still concerned that your milk flow is not adequate for your newborn. A little education and practice will most often relieve your concerns, enabling you to enjoy the primordial mammalian experience of nourishing your offspring.

Feeding Time

Make feeding time a consciously intimate and loving experience. Whether you are breast- or bottle-feeding, cuddle your baby close to your body with her belly toward your belly while you feed her. Make eye contact and send thoughts of love and appreciation to the new soul that has been entrusted into your care. While feeding your baby, bring your awareness fully into the process by closing your eyes and breathing slowly. Feel your arms around your baby as you embrace her. Notice your belly rising and falling against her body. Feel her molding into you. Sense her head in your arms and be aware of her tiny hands touching you. Experience your love and care flowing through you as you nourish her.

Relieving Breast Fullness or Engorgement

To relieve breast fullness, try more frequent feedings for a time. Vary your breastfeeding positions so all areas of your breasts can be drained. Apply warm compresses before feedings and cold compresses after feedings for comfort or stand in a warm shower several times a day. Gently massage your breast with strokes moving from the periphery to the nipple. Make certain that your bra fits properly and you are not irritating your breast with heavy bags or purses.

If despite the measures above, your breasts remain excessively sore, or you are having a fever, contact your health professional. If an antibiotic is prescribed, be certain that it is safe for use during breastfeeding. Gingerroot, chamomile, or calendula soaks can provide symptomatic relief.

Life Force–Enhancing Exercises for Parents

Caring for your baby provides the opportunity to rediscover the world. Seeing the universe through the eyes of your baby can be a precious reminder that life is magical and miraculous. To recapture the wonder that you experienced as a child, take time each day to tune into the five natural elements in the world—earth, air, fire, water, and space. These life force–enhancing suggestions will nourish your newborn baby and your own inner child.

- Weather permitting, walk barefoot on the earth for at least ten minutes each day. Have your attention on your feet with the intention to absorb nourishment from Mother Earth.
- Walk along natural bodies of water, allowing the cooling, cleansing, coherent influence of water to infuse your being.
- Allow the light and warmth of the sun to permeate you. Acknowledge the energy-giving force of the sun, the source of all life on earth.
- Take a walk where there is abundant vegetation and deeply inhale the breath of plants. The ideal time to receive the life force of plants is at dawn and dusk.
- Gaze into the stars at night. Allow your awareness to fill the heavens and the cosmos to fill your awareness.
- Eat locally grown, fresh, and lovingly prepared fruits, vegetables, and grains, which imbibe the life force of all five elements.

Nurturing Your Baby

A new story begins with the birth of your baby. The nine months of pregnancy during which you cared for your child by caring for yourself set the stage for a magical beginning. As you tenderly care for your baby over the next few months, ensure that the love and support that began in your womb continues to flow. This new life has been entrusted into your protection so that her physical, emotional, and spiritual needs are attended. Pay attention to nourishing all of your baby's senses. Have sweet sounds, tender touches, interesting and beautiful visual stimuli, nourishing tastes, and soothing aromas available for your baby to enjoy. Along with your love and care, these nurturing sounds, sensations, sights, flavors, and smells will provide your baby with the building blocks for a healthy, enriched, and enchanted life.

Your Baby's Flow of Consciousness

Research by Boston-based Dr. Peter Wolf, a child psychiatrist, and Dutch psychologist Heinz Prechtl has outlined and elaborated the six different states of consciousness that a newborn baby experiences. Being aware of these states enables you to better understand and respond to your baby's needs throughout the day. The six states of awareness are quiet alertness, active alertness, drowsiness, quiet sleep, active sleep, and crying.

During her *quiet alert state*, your baby is responsive and focuses on you when you talk to her. Her body is relaxed and her eyes are alert. Your baby is very receptive in this state, and it is a wonderful time to deepen your bond with your newborn.

During the *active alert state*, your baby demonstrates rhythmic body movements, which seem to be her way of interacting with you as you communicate with her. She will be interested in looking around at her surroundings while she is in this state, but may not be as interested in making eye contact with you.

Your baby will enter into the *drowsy state* as she awakens or falls off to sleep. Although her eyes may open and close, she will not be focusing on anything in particular. Her eyelids will begin to sag as she drifts off and you may even see her eyes roll upward while her lids are still partially open. She is in the state between wakefulness and sleep.

During *quiet sleep* your baby's face and body will be relaxed with very little movement. Her breathing will be peaceful, although she may sigh periodically.

Active sleep is the baby's equivalent of REM (rapid eye movements) sleep in adults. Your baby will be asleep but physically active in this state. She may wiggle and move, make silly faces, and have periods of sucking. She may even scoot her body close to you for warmth while staying asleep in this state.

Crying is your baby's way of letting you know that she needs something. She may need food, warmth, or comfort. You can usually soothe her in this state by feeding her, picking her up, or cuddling with her. Crying is a form of communication for babies. She may be telling you she is uncomfortable or simply wants to know that you are close by. As you lovingly respond to her cries, she will learn to trust that you are listening and caring for her needs.

Baby Talk

Babies have many ways of relating to you and the world. They cry, fuss, wiggle, kick, listen, stare, change their expressions, look into your eyes, and smile. They are continually learning how to communicate their needs to you through their movements and sounds. Your baby may seem to be in conversation with you as she learns to converse by watching your facial expressions and imitating them back to you. She continues to dialogue as she learns to move her body in synchronized movements to the inflections in your voice.

There is always a reason when your baby cries. She may want to be fed, cuddled, comforted, or changed. She may be trying to tell you that she needs help falling asleep. Over the first few months you will learn to accurately interpret your baby's cries and you will become more adept at understanding her unique way of being and communicating.

Sleeping Together

There are many opportunities to bond with your baby. For some it's through co-sleeping, in what has become known in the West as the "family bed." In many cultures throughout the world babies sleep in bed with their parents for their first few months or even years. Bed sharing has been shown to stabilize a baby's heart rate and reduce crying. It also encourages frequent breastfeedings, and has been suggested to reduce the risk of sudden infant death syndrome (SIDS).

There is controversy regarding co-sleeping. Concerns have been raised by the Consumer Products Safety Commission regarding infant deaths every year attributed to accidents as a result of babies sleeping in adult beds. Most often these are due to entrapment of the baby's head in a bed structure, although suffocation from an adult rolling onto the baby is also reported.

Recent studies have found that more people in America are sharing beds with their babies. The percentage of infants and parents co-sleeping rose from 5.5 percent in 1993 to 12.8 percent in 2000. Babies and mothers that sleep together show synchronization in their movement and breathing patterns. Mothers who sleep with their babies are also more attentive, performing protective behaviors such as kissing, touching, and repositioning their infants five times more than when mothers and babies sleep in separate rooms. If, as an expression of your desire to stay close to your baby you decide to share your bed with her, be certain that you take the necessary precautions to prevent accidental injuries by keeping pillows away from your baby's face and removing any structures that could possibly entrap her.

Nurturing Your Baby Through Her Senses

Your baby learns about the world through her senses. Just as you pay attention to the nourishing food she receives through her mouth, attend to your baby's other senses by focusing on nourishing sounds, sensations, sights, and smells. Talk, read, and sing to your baby. Spend time in natural environments where the sounds, sights, and smells of nature can nourish both of you.

NOURISHING SOUNDS

Your baby has been listening to the beat of your heart and the sound of your voice for months before her birth. These familiar rhythms and vibrations are reassuring to her. Holding her against your chest where she can hear your heartbeat and sweetly conversing with her will soothe and comfort your baby.

As you talk and interact with your baby, assume that your new child is an intelligent being. You will naturally find yourself using higher pitched tones, because your baby will show greater responsiveness when you do so. Like most people, babies like to be looked at while they are spoken to. Many studies have confirmed that your baby prefers your voice to any other female voice, and prefers her father's voice to any other male voice.

Exposing your baby to a wide variety of nourishing sounds stimulates neurological development. Listen to different types of music. Sing, read poetry, tell stories. Take regular walks so your baby can enjoy the primordial sounds of nature—birds chirping, water flowing in streams, the wind rustling the leaves of trees. She will soon begin to make sense out of the different sounds, tones, and syllables to which she is exposed.

NOURISHING TOUCH

Many studies have demonstrated the need for infants to receive regular nourishing touch to support healthy emotional and physical development. Keep your baby snuggled up to you as much as possible. She is nurtured by the warmth and closeness of your body. Make your baby's transition from the womb to the world as effortless and stress free as possible.

The skin is the largest sensory organ in the body, and dozens of studies have shown that babies who are lovingly touched have more stable nervous systems, enhanced immune function, and improved digestive systems. Reports from the University of Miami have demonstrated that premature babies in neonatal intensive care units receiving daily massages put on weight faster and are able to leave the hospital sooner. Massage can help ease colic, stimulate circulation, improve sleep, boost immunity, and enhance bonding and attachment. Massaging your baby on a daily basis is a wonderful way to connect with her.

Massaging Your Baby. Trust yourself in intuiting what is good for your baby. Your loving intention is more important than any particular technique. Explore a variety of strokes as you massage the different parts of her body. Discontinue the massage if your baby gets upset, as newborns may only enjoy short periods initially. Go slowly and enjoy this loving space with your baby. The following steps are guidelines for your baby's first massage. Improvise to create a massage that flows well for you.

Preparation. Create a safe and comfortable space for your baby's massage experience. Keep the temperature in the room comfortably warm, for your baby's body is still learning to regulate its temperature. Uncover only the part of your baby that you are massaging. Use only pure natural edible oil, such as sesame, almond, or sunflower.

Make eye contact with your baby as you begin, making certain that this is a good time for a massage. Throughout the massage continue making eye contact while softly talking or singing to her. Newborn babies often keep their arms and legs

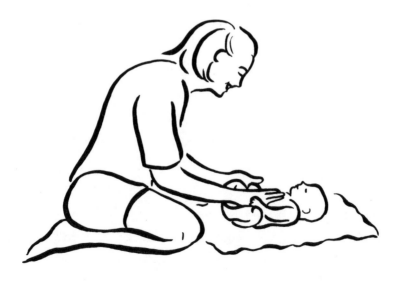

folded closely to their body. Avoid pulling on her limbs, allowing your strokes to glide gently over her flexed arms and legs. The most important principle of a successful massage is that both you and your baby enjoy it.

Feet and Legs. It's often easiest to begin massaging your baby around her feet and legs, which seem to be less sensitive places on her body. Try massaging your baby during a diaper change, while you are getting your baby dressed, or before or after a bath. Use your fingers or whole palm with each stroke.

Begin by uncovering one of your baby's legs and warming a few drops of oil in your hands. Gently massage the top of your baby's thigh and hip with circular motions. Stroke up and down her thigh and then around her knee. Perform up-and-down strokes over her lower leg and then move to her foot. Massage her foot on the top from her toes to her ankle, and then around the bottom of her foot. Massage her little ankle and ankle bones, and then her little toes. If her toes curl up, let them stay curled and massage around them.

If she is calm and enjoying the massage, do the other leg. If she becomes fussy, then begin with the other leg the next time. About the time your baby is six to eight weeks old she will begin to enjoy long strokes down her leg from her hip to her foot.

Buttocks. The buttocks are easy to reach during diaper changes and if allowed by your baby, can follow the massage of her legs. Uncover your baby's buttocks, and with a few drops of warm oil in your hands gently massage your baby's buttocks using small circular motions, one side at a time. To reach her entire buttocks hold your baby to your chest with one hand and massage her lower buttocks with the other hand using circular motions.

Belly. Massaging your baby's belly can help soothe colicky discomfort due to congested gas. Expose your baby's belly, after placing a few drops of oil in your hands. Beginning on the right side of your baby's tummy, massage in small circular clockwise motions spiraling from her navel outward. Avoid getting oil on her healing umbilical cord. Continue massaging in larger and larger circles until you cover the entire abdominal area.

Chest. With a few drops of warm oil on your hands, place your fingers on your baby's chest and glide your hand down along the sides of her torso, bringing your hands together over her belly. Gently cover her chest and sternum as you stroke from her clavicle to her belly, repeating several times.

Arms. New babies often keep their arms flexed close to their body. Do not force your baby to extend her upper arms; rather, gently stroke around her bent joints. Apply a few drops of warm oil in a circular motion around her shoulder, back-and-forth motions over the upper arm, circular over the elbow, back-and-forth over the forearm, circular around her wrist, and gently over each finger.

Back. Your baby will begin strengthening the muscles in her back as she learns to hold her head up and exercises her arms and legs. Massage her back while holding your baby upright against your chest or try laying her facedown over your legs or another soft surface. Using a few drops of warm oil, gently glide your fingers or palm with light pressure along your baby's back from her shoulders down to her buttocks. Repeat this motion several times. Then, starting at the neck, gently make small circular strokes with one or two fingers along each side of the spine down to the lower back. Again, repeat several times from the neck to the sacrum.

Scalp. A gentle scalp massage is comforting and nurturing. It's best to allow the oil on the head to be absorbed for a little while and then shampooed out. Massage your baby's scalp using a small amount of oil over her entire head, as if shampooing her hair, being particularly gentle over the fontanels, or soft spots where the skull bones have not yet come together.

Face. Babies are often sensitive about having their faces touched. Check with your baby to make certain that the experience is enjoyable for her. If she doesn't like it at first, try again in a few weeks. If she seems willing, try starting with your baby's ears, which generates a relaxing feeling throughout the entire body. Next, move to her forehead, using gentle circular motions, and then continue this around her temples. With one or two fingers gently stroke from the forehead along the outer edges of her face down along her jawline to her chin. Repeat this stroke a few times. Because babies are born with a rooting reflex triggered by stimulation on the cheeks and lips, avoid stroking these areas for the first few weeks.

Once you have finished the massage, spend a few minutes holding your baby close to you before dressing or bathing her. Tender touching is one of the most direct ways we have to demonstrate our love to the people in our lives. Taking the time to massage your baby will ensure a magical beginning to her life.

NOURISHING SIGHTS

Infants see best at a distance of about 8 to 10 inches from their eyes and are particularly fascinated by human faces. They tune into various facial expressions and early on begin to imitate them. Most babies are vocalizing by four weeks and smiling responsively by six weeks. They have intense curiosity for their world and a voracious appetite to engage with their environment.

Have colorful, interesting shapes and objects around for your baby to see. She is constantly learning, remembering, and sorting through visual images. Although she will not be able to focus fully for a while, spend time in beautiful, natural settings that nourish all her senses.

NOURISHING SMELLS

Research has shown that your baby is able to recognize your smell within the first couple of days of life. In the brain, smell, memory, and emotion are closely linked. When a smell is initially associated with an experience, the smell alone can later trigger the feelings associated with the original experience. You can use this phenomenon, known as neuro-associative conditioning, to enhance the comfort and well-being of your baby by consciously creating associations between fragrances and comforting experiences. For example, during massage diffuse a soothing aroma, such as lavender, rose, vetiver, or vanilla. Your baby will begin to associate the aroma with a comforting sensation so that in times of discomfort the scent by itself may create a relaxing response.

A SENSE OF HUMOR

Research has shown that laughter may be one of the best medicines. Studies have found that a good belly laugh enhances immune function all day. Make playfulness with your baby a regular part of your daily schedule. By the end of her second month, she will respond to your funny faces and peekaboo games. Remembering to lighten up and not take yourself too seriously is good for both you and your baby.

Nurturing the Nurturer

One of the most important things mothers and father can do to be good parents is to take care of themselves. Once you have established a semblance of rhythm in your new family, ask a close relative or trusted friend to watch your baby for a short while so you can have some time to yourself. Also, make it a priority for you and your spouse or partner to nourish the bond that created your baby. It is not selfish to take care of yourself; rather, it is essential that you maintain your own mind-body balance so you can provide everything your new child needs to flourish physically, emotionally, and spiritually.

Enliven Through Your Attention

• Place your hands on your belly a few times throughout the day and send loving thoughts to your unborn baby.

• Journal each day about your experiences.

• Early in your pregnancy, plant a tree or flowering bush to symbolize the growth of your baby in the womb. After your child is born, you can take care of the plant together.

• Read enchanting stories and heartfelt poetry aloud to your baby and listen to beautiful, relaxing music each day.

• Perform a daily oil massage on yourself before you bathe or shower.

• Diffuse an aroma while listening to music, while soaking in a tub, or while meditating to create the association between the fragrance and the relaxed state of awareness.

• Ensure that you have all six tastes available during your meals throughout the day.

• Choose to eat meals that are rich in color, aroma, and texture.

• Be mindful as you eat your meals. Eat at least one meal each week in silence with your full awareness.

• Practice meditation for twenty to thirty minutes twice daily.

• Pay attention to signals of stress that you experience during the day and employ stress-reducing behaviors to minimize the harmful effects of stress on you and your unborn baby.

• Perform yoga postures with awareness on a regular basis, being gentle and respectful of your body.

• Embrace your pregnancy as an opportunity to experience more natural healing approaches to common minor health concerns.

• Whenever an uncomfortable symptom arises, go through a mental checklist to ensure that you are taking time to relax, eating properly, drinking enough fluids, and exercising regularly.

• Develop an open line of communication with your health care provider and have a low threshold for calling about any emotional or physical concern that may arise.

• Commit to improving your conscious communication skills. When you are feeling upset, determine what you really need and ask for the behavior that will fulfill your need.

• Practice the seven steps for emotional clearing when you are experiencing emotional turbulence. Notice how empowering the process can be when you take responsibility for your feelings.

• Whenever you are finding it difficult to communicate with your partner about your feelings, create the opportunity to practice conscious listening.

• Become familiar with the stages and phases of labor and birth. Knowing the map will increase the likelihood that you get to where you want to go.

• Practice your breathing exercises so you can draw upon a wide range of centering techniques during labor.

• Explore with your birthing partner various massage, pressure, and breathing practices so you can build confidence that he will be there for you when you need his assistance.

• Commit to taking it very easy for the first few weeks after birthing your baby. Make bonding with your newborn your highest priority.

• Take care of your perineum and bottom, using sitz baths and herbal packs to reduce swelling and discomfort.

• Use all five senses to connect with your baby and create a nurturing environment for both of you.

CHAPTER 9

Fatherhood Fundamentals

It is a wise father that knows his own child.

—WILLIAM SHAKESPEARE

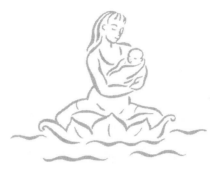

*W*ith the birth of your child, the stuff you are made of passes into the next generation. From a purely genetic perspective your life is deemed successful simply by passing on your DNA, but as a human father, you have deep drives to be an active force in the rearing of your child. More than ever before there is the need and the opportunity for dads to be essential participants in the parenting of healthy and happy children.

You may or may not have had good modeling for an engaged father as you were growing up, but as the late Dr. Benjamin Spock once said, "The more people have studied different methods of bringing up children the more they have come to the conclusion that what good mothers and fathers instinctively feel like doing for their babies is the best after all." In other words, if you are tuned into your inner voice, you will be a good parent to your children.

From the moment you learn that your wife is pregnant, your life begins transforming. As more and more of her attention goes inward to her developing baby, your role as nurturer and supporter expands. The rapidity of physical, emotional, and spiritual changes your wife goes through during pregnancy is on a different scale than most men will ever experience in their own bodies and minds. At times the ride is exhilarating and at times daunting, but be assured that since the beginning of humanity, the course of the next nine months has been successfully traversed by generations of men before you.

Over the next nine months the focus of your life will be on your wife and your developing baby. The promise of a new child rallies the love and attention of people in your life. Intense feelings are the norm rather than the exception for both you and your wife during this initial period, and you need to expect ups and downs as you navigate this new experience together. Let's focus on what you can do physically, emotionally, and spiritually to maintain your balance as your world changes.

Caring for Your Body

It is nearly as important for you to care for yourself as it is for the mother of your child-to-be. Successful parenting requires stamina, and taking care of your own health will enable you to be in a better position to support your wife and your baby. Pay attention to the basics:

- good nutrition
- regular exercise
- stress management
- sound sleep

NUTRITION

Feed your body with nourishing food. Balanced nutrition does not have to be complex, but you do need to put attention on ingesting a wide variety of foods to receive the nutrients that keep you healthy and vital. Following a diet rich in six tastes and seven colors enables you to metabolize the health-promoting intelligence of nature into the healthy chemistry and physiology of your body. To cover your nutritional bases, we also encourage you to take a high-potency multiple vitamin for its long-term health promoting benefits.

If you are not already accomplished at cooking, this is a good time to learn. Learning to cook will enhance your sense of self-sufficiency and provide another opportunity for you to support your wife and baby. Pick up a couple of cookbooks and practice preparing some wholesome recipes. Being able to multitask will be good for the entire family.

EXERCISE

You need to maintain your physical fitness. The benefits of exercise are on multiple levels, ranging from reducing stress to improving sleep. Although exercise time is often one of the first things to be left out when life becomes demanding, we encourage you to make it a high priority.

There are three primary components to a balanced exercise program: flexibility, strength training, and cardiovascular conditioning. Each of these approaches enhances both physical and emotional well-being. Many studies support the value of exercise in lowering anxiety levels, raising the production of natural antidepressants, and reducing anger and irritability. In addition to feeling stronger and having better aerobic capacity, the mood-stabilizing benefits of exercise will serve you well over the next nine months.

Set your fitness regimen and stick with it. If possible, do something physical every day. An ideal program would be to perform ten minutes of yoga or other stretching exercise followed by strength training for twenty minutes three days per week and cardiovascular conditioning for twenty minutes three days per week. On the seventh day, take a leisurely walk with your spouse.

STRESS MANAGEMENT

It's natural to feel some anxiety when a new baby is on the way. Your life is undergoing changes over which you have very limited control. The added financial responsibilities of a new member of the family may naturally create some concern. Learning to manage your stress will help you make the most successful decisions to maintain your balance.

Take time to quiet your mind in meditation daily. Practice a mindfulness technique, learn a mantra, or listen to meditation tapes. For over thirty years, studies have shown that people who experience restful awareness through meditation regularly are emotionally and physically healthier. Remember, you are of greatest benefit to your family when you are coming from a centered and calm place within yourself.

SOUND SLEEP

Your body needs sleep to rejuvenate. If you do not get the rest you need each night, you accumulate fatigue, which impairs your ability to stay centered in the midst of challenges. Studies have shown that inadequate rest results in immune weakness, lowered pain thresholds, impaired concentration, and poorer memory recall. According to Ayurveda, sleep is the nursemaid to humanity and one of the pillars of health.

To the best of your ability, try to follow an ideal daily routine that includes rising with the sun, meditating in the morning, exercising for half an hour, taking time at midday to eat a nourishing lunch, meditating a second time before your lighter evening meal, and getting to bed no later than 10:30 p.m. If you are having trouble falling asleep because you have too much on your mind, try the following simple sleep routine.

• Run a hot bath an hour before bedtime, adding a few drops of calming aromatherapy oil such as lavender, sandalwood, or vanilla to the water.

• Perform a slow oil massage on yourself while the bath is running. (See the massage description in Chapter 2, page 54.)

• After your massage, soak in the warm tub for ten to fifteen minutes.

• After your bath, drink a cup of warm milk with nutmeg and honey, or some chamomile or valerian root tea.

• Journal for a few minutes before bed, "downloading" your concerns so you are not ruminating about them when you shut your eyes.

• Read mind-quieting literature for a few minutes before bed, avoiding dramatic novels or distressing material.

• Avoid watching television or doing mind-activating work in bed.

• Once in bed, close your eyes and bring your attention into your body. Wherever you notice tension, consciously relax that area, then simply watch your slow, easy breathing until you fall asleep.

If you are lying still in bed quietly observing your breath, your metabolic activity is nearly as low as if you were in deep sleep. Even if your mind is still awake, your body is getting the rest it needs. Therefore, do not worry if you are not immediately falling asleep, and by not worrying, you will quickly drift off into a deep slumber.

Overcoming Emotional Turbulence

As a father-to-be you need to acknowledge that you cannot fully understand or appreciate what your pregnant wife or partner is going through. Her body is changing on a daily basis and the hormonal fluxes that are occurring inside her can contribute to rapid emotional shifts. Add these physiological and biochemical changes to her natural anxieties about pregnancy, birth, and mothering and you have the recipe for an occasional emotional meltdown. Compassion for your spouse is a useful quality to mobilize when occasionally she does not seem like her usual stable self. It's important that you not take her emotional perturbations too personally, but, rather, look for opportunities to provide support and balance.

Your spouse wants and needs your unconditional love and nurturing as she experiences the physical and emotional turbulence of pregnancy. This means being willing to relinquish your attachment to rigid ideas about what you believe she should think or feel about her changing world. Intellectual analysis will usually not be of much help in navigating the emotional turbulence of pregnancy. Pregnancy is an opportunity to be a true spiritual warrior, cultivating flexibility without weakness, patience without negligence, and acceptance without resignation.

When your spouse is upset, remember that her distress is the result of a need that is not being met. Whether or not she is expressing her need in a fully conscious way, see if you can look beyond the emotion to the implied request. Sometimes you will be capable of meeting her needs, and other times you won't, but the more centered you remain, the better you'll be able to help her regain her balance. No one is expected to be perfect—neither you nor your partner—but try to seek creative solutions to the inevitable challenges that arise.

Review the principles of conscious communication developed in Chapter 6. Although ideally both partners consistently differentiate their observations and feelings from their judgments and interpretations, it is easy to fall back into a pattern of holding the other person responsible for your feelings during periods of emotional turbulence. Resist becoming engaged in emotional battles of attack and defend. Rather, identify what it is that actually happened, acknowledge the feelings that were triggered by the situation, uncover the need that was not met, and offer the behavior that will fulfill the need.

Your role as a supporting spouse is to maximize the safety, security, and stability in your wife's life, knowing that this is the greatest value you can provide to your unborn child. Before engaging in conflict and confrontation, consider that your unborn baby is on the receiving end of the strong uncomfortable feelings that are generated. You wouldn't have a heated argument with your newborn baby, so do your best to avoid one with your wife.

If despite your best efforts, the immediate stresses lead to an emotionally charged encounter, try to dissipate the strong feelings and resolve the conflict as quickly as possible. When you feel yourself getting emotionally overloaded and losing your center, practice the seven steps of emotional processing to regain your composure. Let's take an example of a common scenario to see how this might work.

> *Driving home from a day at the office you get caught in rush-hour traffic and arrive at your house twenty minutes later than you had planned. Unfortunately, you forgot that your wife had a pregnancy yoga class she wanted to attend. Because you were supposed to be home in time to watch your three-year-old son, she is now at risk of missing her class. She is irritated and unloads on you about how selfish and irresponsible you are.*

This encounter could easily go one way or the other. On one hand, it would not take much for you to react to her attack by taking out your frustrations on her over your stressful day and challenging commute home. However, engaging in a reactive response will only lead to more hurt feelings on both sides and possibly prolong the period before reconciliation, an approach that is not best for you, your spouse, or your unborn baby.

Alternatively, we encourage you to try a different tactic.

Instead of mobilizing your psychological defenses, recognize that as a result of the discrepancy between the time you were expected to arrive and the time you showed up, your wife experienced strong feelings of frustration, disappointment, irritation, and anxiety. She has a need to attend her class, and the fulfillment of that need is in jeopardy. Rather than reacting to her reaction, simply say, "I'm really sorry I'm late. I didn't leave enough time to account for the terrible traffic. I promise from now on when you want to go to your class, I will allow for extra time to drive home. Why don't you leave right now for your class, and we can talk more about this later?"

Both your wife's and your upset feelings are legitimate. However, at this time in her life it is especially important not to engage in a vehement argument. Once she is on her way to her class, sit for a few minutes and tune into the sensations in your body. Allow yourself to feel the strong emotions that have been generated and breathe into them. See if you can identify your feelings without using language that puts you into the role of a victim. Then do something active to release the pressure in your body that your feelings are creating: put your three-year-old into a jogging stroller and go for a twenty-minute run; put on some rock and roll music and vigorously straighten up the house; move your body with the intention to release the impulse to fight or run.

By the time your wife arrives home, you'll be in a much better state of mind to discuss the incident without escalating the issue to an argument. Your commitment to minimizing the violence in your life is good for you, your partner, and your baby-to-be. Developing these healthy patterns will serve you well as your family grows. Your children's style of communication is shaped long before they are capable of intellectually analyzing how they relate to the world. Help them establish healthy principles early on that will help them meet their emotional needs throughout their lives.

Awakening Your Spirit

According to Ayurveda, human beings have four basic needs in life: *artha*, *kama*, *dharma*, and *moksha*. Becoming a parent provides motivation and opportunity for you to meet each of these needs.

Artha means "things." People naturally aspire to own things and derive pleasure from a healthy measure of material abundance. When you have children, it is natural to desire a comfortable home, a safe automobile, and adequate resources to provide for your children's needs. On the other hand, if you expend all your energy on the acquisition of wealth, your financial assets may increase, but the other important components of your life will suffer. Manage your resources responsibly, strive for abundance, but never let it alienate you from your loved ones. No one at the time of their death ever regrets that they did not go into work earlier or stay later at the office.

Kama refers to love in all its expressions, including sensual love. We have an inherent need to connect intimately with people in our lives. Nourishing relationships are essential to healthy and fulfilling lives. A basic theme of this book has been to encourage you to make nurturing relationships the highest priority in your family. If your relationships are loving, you can weather all challenges in your life. Practice love in your life and teach love to your children. It is one of the most important responsibilities you have to maximize their potential for happy and successful lives.

Dharma means living in accordance with the laws of nature. According to the law of dharma, people are born with a unique set of talents, which when developed enables them to make a contribution to their community, while generating the artha, or material abundance they require to live comfortably. One of the most important roles that parents play is to help their children cultivate their special talents. Expose your children to as wide a range of experiences as possible and observe those opportunities to which they are naturally attracted or in which they excel. If your child shows talent in an area, encourage and support him, rather than imposing your idea about how he should be living his life. When people are in their dharma, they tend to lose track of time. Timeless awareness is one of the best signs that a person is living in accordance with their soul's purpose in life.

Finally, *moksha* means "liberation." According to Ayurveda the ultimate goal of life is liberating your soul through the transformation of your internal reference point from ego to spirit. Moksha implies that your self-identity expands in widening circles, so that you identify yourself less and less with your country, religion, ethnic background, or occupation, and increasingly as a sentient, spiritual being. As you expand your identity from local to nonlocal, your capacity for compassion also expands. Your actions become increasingly evolutionary and it becomes impossible to harm another being. Synchronicity and spontaneous fulfillment of your desires become commonplace, while your very presence generates peace, harmony, laughter, and love in those around you. Teaching your children these spiritual principles is our best chance for creating a world that is fit for them to live in.

Stand by Your Woman

While in most situations we are enthusiastic proponents of relationships based upon equality, during pregnancy the equation indisputably shifts in favor of your wife's needs over your own. From the moment you discover she is pregnant until months after birth, we encourage you to be there for her, even when it means deferring gratification of your own needs. There are several important milestone events during the pregnancy when your support is critical and your presence should be your highest priority. At a minimum these include:

- the performance of the pregnancy test
- the first several health care provider visits

- any and all ultrasound studies
- any health care provider visit when there is a concern
- all birth-education classes
- preliminary visits to the hospital or birthing center
- any test procedures
- any health care provider visit when the results of tests are discussed
- the birth

Be intimately involved in the pregnancy and birth of your baby. Your participation at significant moments will deepen your connection to your wife and your unborn child. These events are important and fleeting; if you miss them, you miss a precious opportunity to share in the development and birth of your child. You will never regret the time you take to be deeply engaged in this wondrous process.

Dos and Don'ts

For the sake of peace and harmony in your household, we offer a few suggestions that will serve any potential father well. Remember that your wife or partner is a somewhat different person than she was before becoming pregnant. There are now two people living in her body, and her reactions to you may be different than they have been in the past. People respond differently under stress than they do when they feel completely safe and secure. Stress is common during times of rapid change, and there are few periods in life where change occurs as rapidly as during the nine months of pregnancy.

• Avoid expressing concerns about your wife's changing body shape. Saying anything approaching "Do you think you should be gaining this much weight?" is treading on dangerous ground. Trust that your wife's body is going through the important changes it needs to in order to support your unborn child. In time, after birth, she will return to the shape you remember. Enjoy her voluptuousness now and look for every opportunity to express your appreciation for her beautiful pregnant body.

• If your wife expresses concerns about the appearance of her body, be supportive but do not suggest that you have been worrying about the same thing. If she wonders out loud if the stretch marks are going to be permanent, simply reassure her that they will improve after the baby is born. If she expresses anxiety about whether her belly or breasts will be permanently changed by the pregnancy, reassure her that her body will recover its prior shape in time. Do not say, "I've been wondering the same thing," if you want to preserve peace in your household. Remember, your most important role now is to help reduce, not compound, her worries.

• Be prepared for fluctuations in your wife's sexual appetite. Pregnant women often find their sexual desire ebbing and flowing. It is not uncommon for women to have little desire during the first trimester due to a combination of physical and emotional factors. If your wife is struggling with morning sickness, it shouldn't surprise you that her interest in passionate love making moves to the back burner.

During the second trimester, women often experience the return of a healthy sexual appetite. The blood engorgement in your partner's sexual organs enhances her sensitivity and pleasure. This is an opportunity to experiment with different positions that do not place uncomfortable pressure on her expanding womb.

By the time she is in her third trimester, your partner's sexual enthusiasm will probably be waning. Carrying an enlarging baby is increasingly hard work and it is difficult for her to feel comfortable in her body. It is certainly possible to enjoy safe and pleasurable sex at this stage; you'll simply need to be more sensitive and creative. Remember, even if you are not engaging in intercourse, you can still be affectionate and sensual with each other. Follow her lead and try not to take her lack of sexual passion personally.

• Make your choices bearing in mind the possibility that everything may not unfold exactly as planned. When it is time to go to a pregnancy checkup with her, leave enough time so you are not late due to unanticipated delays. Allow enough time until your next professional appointment so you will not feel pressure if the visit runs later than expected. Do not plan a business trip out of town within one month of her due date. Do everything in your power to avoid contributing to her anxiety. Letting your spouse know that being there for her is your highest priority will avoid unnecessary conflict.

• Identify someone with whom you can communicate, when it is clear that your issues and concerns are best not brought to the attention of your wife. Your father, brother, or best friend might be a good choice. Establish your own relationship with your wife's doctor or pregnancy advisor and ask him or her the questions that are on your mind. Reassurance that your concerns are normal and easily addressed will keep you in your centered state of being, in which you are of greatest value to your partner and unborn baby.

First Impressions

There is no joy in the world that compares with meeting your child for the first time. Increasingly, fathers are given the opportunity to receive the baby as it emerges from the birth canal. After handing him to your wife, you may also be given the opportunity to cut the umbilical cord. If you have been taking pictures during labor and birth, ask someone else to hold the camera during the final moments of birthing so you can be fully present as your child enters the world. Life can be challenging, but holding your newborn baby at the very beginning of his life makes everything worthwhile at that sacred moment.

There is usually a period after birth—during which the placenta is delivered or tears may need suturing—that you can use to bond with your new baby. The child is often in a state of quiet alertness in which he will be very receptive. Speak to him; sing to him; welcome him into your family and into your heart. This is the beginning of a life-long love affair. You are your baby's father. It is one of the most important and potentially rewarding roles you will ever play. Savor it from the magical beginning.

Enliven Through Your Attention

FOR THE FATHER

- Take care of your own body, mind, and spirit so you can be more available to your wife and new child.
- Flow with the inevitable emotional and physical changes your partner is going through during the pregnancy. Look for opportunities to provide your support.
- Identify your own support systems that you can rely on when you are feeling depleted or overwhelmed.

FOR THE MOTHER

- Place your hands on your belly a few times throughout the day and send loving thoughts to your unborn baby.
- Journal each day about your experiences.
- Early in your pregnancy, plant a tree or flowering bush to symbolize the growth of your baby in the womb. After your child is born, you can take care of the plant together.
- Read enchanting stories and heartfelt poetry aloud to your baby and listen to beautiful, relaxing music each day.

• Perform a daily oil massage on yourself before you bathe or shower.

• Diffuse an aroma while listening to music, while soaking in a tub, or while meditating to create the association between the fragrance and the relaxed state of awareness.

• Ensure that you have all six tastes available during your meals throughout the day.

• Choose to eat meals that are rich in color, aroma, and texture.

• Be mindful as you eat your meals. Eat at least one meal each week in silence with your full awareness.

• Practice meditation for twenty to thirty minutes twice daily.

• Pay attention to signals of stress that you experience during the day and employ stress-reducing behaviors to minimize the harmful effects of stress on you and your unborn baby.

• Perform yoga postures with awareness on a regular basis, being gentle and respectful of your body.

• Embrace your pregnancy as an opportunity to experience more natural healing approaches to common minor health concerns.

• Whenever an uncomfortable symptom arises, go through a mental checklist to ensure that you are taking time to relax, eating properly, drinking enough fluids, and exercising regularly.

• Develop an open line of communication with your health care provider and have a low threshold for calling about any emotional or physical concern that may arise.

- Commit to improving your conscious communication skills. When you are feeling upset, determine what you really need and ask for the behavior that will fulfill your need.

- Practice the seven steps for emotional clearing when you are experiencing emotional turbulence. Notice how empowering the process can be when you take responsibility for your feelings.

- Whenever you are finding it difficult to communicate with your partner about your feelings, create the opportunity to practice conscious listening.

- Become familiar with the stages and phases of labor and birth. Knowing the map will increase the likelihood that you get to where you want to go.

- Practice your breathing exercises so you can draw upon a wide range of centering techniques during labor.

- Explore with your birthing partner various massage, pressure, and breathing practices so you can build confidence that he will be there for you when you need his assistance.

- Commit to taking it very easy for the first few weeks after birthing your baby. Make bonding with your newborn your highest priority.

- Take care of your perineum and bottom, using sitz baths and herbal packs to reduce swelling and discomfort.

- Use all five senses to connect with your baby and create a nurturing environment for both of you.

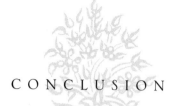

CONCLUSION

*Healing the World
One Child at a Time*

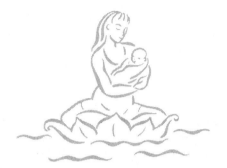

*I*n this book we have given you very practical ways to consciously nurture the life force in your body from the moment of conception. We hope you will utilize these approaches so that your new family will be a beacon of peace, harmony, and love that inspires others in your community to follow your example.

For us, there is a deeper meaning and purpose in writing this book. We have spent decades of our lives studying the ancient wisdom traditions of the world. We have been most influenced by the great healing tradition of Ayurveda, which holds that a human being embodies the most creative expression of the universe in evolution. We are the instruments through which the universe has chosen to be self-conscious. With the birth of every child, the universe chooses to look at itself with fresh eyes. Although you may believe that you look out at the world through your sensory apparatus, the deeper reality is that you are an outcropping of universal intelligence looking at itself through your senses. The Upanishads declare, "*Yatha pinde, tatha brahmande,*" which translated into English reads,

> As is the atom, so is the universe.
> As is the microcosm, so is the macrocosm.
> As is the human body, so is the cosmic body.
> As is the human mind, so is the cosmic mind.

We are at a critical period at this moment in evolutionary time. The predatory instinct survives in us and frequently dominates. At the same time, our deep creative impulses impel us to participate in the harmonious interaction of elements and forces in the cosmos, inspiring us to take the next evolutionary step. The choice is ours. As predators we can ravage the planet, causing the extinction of other species in the web of life, ultimately risking our own extinction. As creators, we can participate in the next evolutionary expression of cosmic intelligence.

The world we see "out there" is our creation. If we have wars, it is because we have agreed to use violence as a means to settle our differences. Ecological devastation, crime, economic disparities, cruelty to animals, and violence in all its forms are the consequence of human choices. The seeds of these destructive impulses reside within each of us, precipitating into collective expressions that are played out locally and globally as acts of terror, tyranny, and environmental pollution.

But we must not forget that even the worst terrorist, tyrant, or polluter was once a child. Each child arrives as a gift from the universe. The wisdom tradition of Vedanta holds that death and birth are interwoven creative acts of the soul. When the physical body gets to the point when it can no longer creatively express the innate wisdom of the soul, the soul goes into incubation in the nonlocal domain, beyond the dimensions of space and time. After a period of incubation, the soul takes a quantum creative leap, choosing to be born again to express its latent potentials, developed over eons of experience.

Love is all that's needed for a new soul to blossom. With loving nurturing the soul finds its next creative expression. But if this loving nurturing is denied, an imbalance between the forces of creativity and inertia results in wounded individuals and a wounded planet. We hope that by embracing the principles in this book, you will make a deep commitment to restoring balance in your own life, while creating an atmosphere of love and nurturing for your child and your family.

We also hope that you will recognize the deep connection between your family, the human family, and the planet as a whole. The future of our planet depends upon who our children become as adults, and it is our responsibility to teach and share with them awareness of the divine intelligence that is the source and sustainer of all life. In *The Prophet*, Kahlil Gibran says,

Your children are not your children.
They are the sons and daughters of Life's longing for itself . . .

The souls of our children are the potential for tomorrow's world. Our earth is not just a capricious anomaly in the vast sea of space, but a cosmic manifestation of divine intelligence. Through leaps of imagination, it will continue to express itself as new realities. Our job as parents is not to interfere with this creative process, but to align with it by nurturing our children in body, mind, and spirit. The great Indian poet Tagore once said, "Every child that is born is proof that God has not yet given up on human beings." We ask you to join with us and with God to help create a world of peace, harmony, laughter, and love that is worthy of our beloved children.

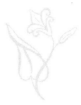

Glossary of Terms

amniotic fluid The fluid within the sac that surrounds the baby in utero

Apgar score An evaluation of the baby's health at one and five minutes after birth

aromatherapy Using the scents of flowers and plants for their effects on the physiology

bearing-down reflex A reaction to the pressure of the baby on the pelvic floor, which causes a spontaneous urge to push

bloody show A blood-tinged mucus discharge, or "mucus plug," which indicates labor is imminent

bonding   The natural attachment that develops between parents and child

Braxton Hicks contractions   Nonprogressive contractions that feel like menstrual cramps

breath awareness   The practice of consciously directing the breath

breathing techniques   *cleansing breath, rhythmic breath, hee breath,* and *blow breath*

breech presentation   When the baby is positioned feet- or bottom-first at the time of delivery

catheter   A tube used for injecting or evacuating fluids, e.g., a urinary catheter or an epidural catheter

cephalopelvic disproportion (CPD)   A relative disproportion of the baby's head to the mother's pelvis; i.e., the baby's head is too large for the birth canal

cervix   The necklike opening of the uterus

cesarean section   A surgical procedure to deliver a baby through openings made in the abdominal wall and uterus

colic   cramping in the abdomen caused by gas in the intestines

colostrum   The first milk secreted by the breasts after giving birth

comfort measures   Steps taken in labor to maximize comfort

consciousness   The continuity of awareness that underlies the mind and the body

contraction   The shortening and thickening of a muscle

crowning   The appearance of the baby's head at the opening of the vagina

delivery accessory bag   Items collected to make the birthing environment more comfortable

dilation   The opening of the cervix in labor

effacement   The softening and thinning of the cervix

epidural   A regional anesthetic that is administered into a spinal space in the lower back

episiotomy   An incision made at the back of the vaginal opening to surgically widen the birth passage

failure to progress   The condition in which labor contractions are inadequate to move the baby toward delivery

fetal distress   A rise or fall in the fetal heart rate that indicates the baby is not receiving enough oxygen

fontanels   The soft, boneless areas in the skull of a young baby that later fuse together

forceps   Two spoon-shaped instruments that are applied to the sides of a baby's head to assist in the delivery process

ghee   Clarified butter

herpes simplex   An infectious disease caused by the herpes virus

IV drip   Intravenous infusions given to the laboring woman to prevent dehydration

life force   The biological energy that sustains the physiological functions of the body

lightening   A sensation that the baby is dropping lower in the pelvis

lochia   The flow of blood and tissue from the vagina after a baby is born

mandala   A visual diagram that brings the attention inward

mantra   A sound that brings coherence to the mind

mindfulness meditation   The practice of observing the flow of breath, which facilitates the quieting of the mind

narcotic   A drug that relieves pain by stimulating the brain's opiate receptors

natural childbirth   Delivery of a baby without the use of medications or other medical interventions

nesting urge   A sudden burst of energy or desire to prepare for the baby's arrival that may occur in early labor

neti pot   A small ceramic kettle filled with warm salted water used to drain excess mucus from the sinuses

paradigm   A model or example; a way of viewing something

pelvic floor toners   Exercises to tone and strengthen the pelvic floor muscles; also called Kegel exercises

perineal massage Lubricating and stretching the vaginal tissues prior to delivery to increase their elasticity

perineum The space surrounding the vagina and the rectum

Pitocin A synthesized hormone given intravenously to induce or accelerate labor

placenta The spongy, blood-rich organ that is attached to the inside wall of the uterus through which the baby is nourished

placental abnormalities A condition wherein the placenta is not appropriately positioned or is at risk of separating prematurely

prolapse The moving out of place or falling of an internal organ

rupture of membranes Breaking the bag of amniotic fluid that surrounds the fetus

Stage I labor The time period from the onset of labor until the cervix fully dilates

Stage II labor The time period from full cervical dilation until the baby is delivered

Stage III labor The time period after the baby is delivered until the delivery of the placenta

timing of contractions The time between the beginning of one contraction to the beginning of the next

transition The stage of labor when the cervix is nearing full dilation and contractions are intense and occurring closer together

trimester   A period of three months within a pregnancy

umbilical cord   The cord that connects the baby to the placenta

uterine massage   A gentle massage given to the postpartum woman's lower abdomen

vacuum extraction   Using an instrument that attaches by suction to the baby's scalp to help ease the baby through the birth canal

welcoming ritual   A loving act performed by the parents immediately after the birth of their child to honor his or her arrival in the world

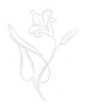

Suggested Reading

Bower, T.G.R. *Development in Infancy*. San Francisco: Freeman, 1974.

Chopra, Deepak, David Simon, and Leanne Backer. *The Chopra Center Cookbook*. New York: John Wiley & Sons, 2002.

Goodlin, Robert C. "The Fetus as a Person (or the Importance of Maternal Tranquility)" in *Care of the Fetus*. New York: Masson Publishing, 1979.

Heber, David. *What Color Is Your Diet?* New York: Regan Books, 2001.

Lieberman, M. Quoted by L.W. Sontag in "Parental Determinants of Postnatal Behavior" in *Fetal Growth and Development*, by H.A. Weisman and G.R. Kerr. New York: McGraw-Hill, 1970.

Marshall, Connie. *From Here to Maternity*. Minden, Nev.: Marshall Educational Health Solutions, 1994.

Miller, Dr. Light, and Dr. Bryan Miller. *Ayurveda & Aromatherapy.* Twin Lakes, Wis.: Lotus Press, 1995.

Murkoff, Heidi E., Arlene Eisenberg, and Sandee E. Hathaway. *What to Expect When You're Expecting.* New York: Workman Publishing, 2002.

Rosenberg, Marshall. *Nonviolent Communication.* Encinitas, Cal.: PuddleDancer Press, 2000.

Samuels, Mike, and Nancy Samuels. *The New Well Pregnancy Book.* New York: Fireside, 1996.

Verny, M.D., Thomas, and John Kelly. *The Secret Life of the Unborn Child.* New York: Dell Publishing, 1981.

Wirsen, Claes, and Lennart Nilsson. *A Child Is Born.* New York: Dell Publishing, 1966.

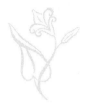

Index

acupressure
   for nausea, 135–36
   to stimulate labor, 221–23
acupuncture, 221–23
Agni, 23
alfalfa, 253
aloe vera, 242–43, 245
amino acids, 84, 85
amniotic fluid, 30, 32, 33, 39–40
anesthesia, epidural, 221,
   224–25
anise, 252–53
appetite, 83–84, 92, 239–40, 253
aromas, *see* smelling and aromas
aroma warm pack, 207–8
artha, 164, 285
asparagus, 253

astringent foods, 76, 79–80
Ayurveda, 8, 45, 49, 184–85,
   239, 297–98
   appearance of life in, 23
   breastfeeding and, 253
   diet and six primary tastes in,
      32, 74, 75, 76–80, 253
   flame of awareness in, 23
   four basic needs in, 164,
      285–87
   fragrances in, 66
   massage in, 55, 57
   nutrition in, 63
   primordial cells in, 20
   sleep in, 279
   Vata, Pitta, and *Kapha*
      imbalances in, 51, 53, 56

baby, newborn, 237–71
   bonding with, 194, 217,
      238–39, 259, 291–92
   breastfeeding of, *see*
      breastfeeding
   communication of, 259
   crying of, 257, 258, 259
   life force-enhancing
      suggestions for, 255–56
   massaging of, 261–68
   nurturing of, 256–57, 261–68
   senses and, 261–68
   sleeping with, 259–60
   states of consciousness of,
      257–58
baby, unborn, 5, 6, 7
   development of, 19–41
   developmental milestones of,
      36–38
   emotions and, 5, 6, 7, 28, 97,
      99
   hearing and, 26–29, 50–54
   kicking by, 30, 48, 54, 99, 101
   nutrition and, 75, 82, 83, 84
   sight and, 31–32, 60–62
   smell and, 32–34, 64–67
   stress and, 98–101, 102
   taste and, 32, 33, 62–63
   touch and, 29–31, 54–60
   womb ecology and, 45–69
   yoga and, 30, 31, 124–25
back pain, 142–44
   in labor, easing of, 206–7
   yoga and, 114–15, 122
balance, maintaining, 97
   see also emotions; meditation;
      stress; yoga
balance (vestibular) system,
   29–30
baths and showers, 209
Bendectin, 134
birth, period following, 237–71

bleeding during, 243
bonding with newborn in, 194,
   217, 238–39, 259, 291–92
contractions during, 243–44
depression during, 248–50
emotions during, 247–48
hemorrhoids and, 242, 245–46
Kegel exercises and, 246–47
life force-enhancing
   suggestions for, 255–56
nurturing yourself during, 268
rejuvenation and
   replenishment during,
   239–40
birthing, *see* labor and birthing
birthing ball, 209–10
bitter foods, 76, 79
blastocyst, 22–23, 24
bleeding, postpartum, 243
bonding, 194, 217, 238–39, 259,
   291–92
Bower, T.G.R., 61–62
breastfeeding, 241, 250–55, 260
   colostrum in, 250–51
   contractions and, 243
   feeding time experience in,
      254–55
   herbs to enhance milk supply,
      252–53
   relieving breast fullness, 255
breathing exercises, 197–203
Buddha, 49
butterfly pose, 111–13

calendula, 255
carbohydrates, 76
cat and cow pose, 113–15
Cayce, Edgar, 17
cervix, dilation of, 186, 187, 188
cesarean delivery (c-section),
   221, 224, 227–29

chamomile, 242, 255
changes, physical, 129–50
childbirth, *see* labor and birthing
child's pose, 119–20
Chinese medicine, 57
choice making, 6, 7–8, 68
Chopra Center, 6, 99, 155
chromosomes, 20
cinnamon, 252–53
colors of foods, 75, 80–81
colostrum, 250–51
communication skills
  of babies, 259
  conscious listening, 171–72
  in relationships, 153, 154,
    157–58, 160–68, 169,
    171–72, 282–85, 289
conception, 7, 17, 19–26
constipation, 137–38
contractions, 115, 186–90, 197,
    209, 217, 219, 220–21, 223
  afterbirth, 243–44
  simulating, 190–91
creative imagination, 13–15
crowning, 191

depression, 55, 104
  postpartum, 248–50
dharma, 164, 285, 286
diet, 63, 73–93
  appetite and, 83–84, 92,
    239–40, 253
  colors of foods in, 75, 80–81
  eating with awareness, 88,
    90–91
  expanding enjoyment at meals,
    91–93
  fatherhood and, 277–78
  labor and, 208
  morning sickness and, 131–32,
    133, 136

postpartum, 239–40, 241
  in pregnancy, 82–88, 91–93
  protein in, 76, 77, 80, 84–86
  six primary tastes in, 32, 75,
    76–80, 253
  vegetarian, 85
digestive problems, 129
  constipation, 137–38
  heartburn and indigestion,
    136–37
  morning sickness, 78–79,
    130–36
dim lights, 209
DNA, 4, 20, 75, 275
drawing, 10, 12–13
drugs, 129–30, 132–33
  for pain, 216, 221, 224–25

egg (ovum), 19–22, 36
ego boundaries, 164–65, 169
Emerson, Ralph Waldo, 107
emotions, 153–74
  ambivalent, 154–57
  communication skills and, 153,
    154, 157–58, 160–68, 169,
    282–85, 289
  fatherhood and, 281–85
  mood swings, 144–45, 247
  needs and, 159–61, 164,
    165–68, 169, 282
  peaceful, fostering, 157–58
  postpartum, 247–48
  releasing emotional toxicity,
    169–71
  sensory perception and, 46–47
  unborn baby and, 5, 6, 7, 28,
    97, 99
  vocabulary of, 162–64
  see also stress
endorphins and encephalins, 47,
    187, 216

epidural anesthesia, 221, 224–25
episiotomy, 226–27
essential fatty acids, 75, 77,
    86–87
essential oils, 65–67
estrogen, 25
exercise ball, 209–10
exercises
    fatherhood and, 278
    Kegel, 122–24, 246–47
    yoga, *see* yoga
external fetal monitoring, 219

fat, 76
father (partner), 237, 275–94
    ambivalent emotions and,
        154–57
    bonding and, 239, 291–92
    communication skills and, 153,
        154, 157–58, 160–68, 169,
        171–72, 282–85, 289
    conscious listening and,
        171–72
    dos and don'ts for, 288–91
    emotions and, 281–85
    exercise for, 278
    health care for, 277–81
    labor and, 210–11
    nurturing of, after birth of
        baby, 268
    nutrition for, 277–78
    sleep and, 279–81
    stress management for, 279
    as supporting spouse, 281, 282,
        287–88, 289–90
    voice of, 52, 54, 261
feeling (touch), *see* touch and
    feeling
feelings, *see* emotions
fennel, 252–53
fenugreek, 252

fertilization, 21–22, 36
fetus, *see* baby, unborn
fight-or-flight response, 28, 98, 99,
    197
fish, 86–87
flavors, *see* tasting and flavors
fluid retention, 145–46
folic acid, 88
food, *see* diet
Freud, Sigmund, 154

genes, 3, 20, 22, 275
Gibran, Kahlil, 300
ginger, 78–79, 133–34, 242, 255
glossary of terms, 301–306

health, definition of, 6–7
health care provider, 130,
    147–48
hearing and sounds, 45, 46, 47,
    49, 50–54, 68, 104
    music, *see* music
    newborn and, 241, 257,
        261–62
    postpartum, 241
    in the womb, 26–29, 50–54
heartburn and indigestion,
    136–37
Heber, David, 80
Heidegger, Martin, 50
hemorrhoids, 124, 138–39, 242,
    245–46
herbal ice packs, 241–42
herbs
    for breast soreness, 255
    to enhance milk supply,
        252–53
    for hemorrhoids, 246
    for morning sickness, 134
    for perineal discomfort, 242

for postpartum contractions,
244
hormones, 247
in labor, 189, 192–93, 205,
209, 216–17, 220
oxytocin, 189, 205, 209,
216–17, 220, 223, 243
in pregnancy, 22–23, 113, 145
progesterone, 25, 137, 138
stress and, 28, 47, 48, 98, 103
human chorionic gonadotropin
(hCG), 24–25
humor, 268

ice packs, herbal, 241–42
images, *see* seeing and images
imagination, 13–15
insomnia, 130, 139–40
fatherhood and, 279–81
intelligence of nature, 35–36
intravenous access, 220

Jivaka, 49
Jones, Jamison, 100
journaling, 10–12
juice, 208, 220

Kabir, 105
kama, 164, 285–86
Kapha imbalance, 51, 53, 56
Kegel, Arnold, 246
Kegel exercises, 122–24, 246–47

labor and birthing, 177–233
affirmations for, 215
back pain in, 206–7
bonding with newborn after,
194, 217

breathing exercises for,
197–203
cesarean delivery, 221, 224,
227–29
checklist for, 182–83
contractions in, 115, 186–90,
197, 209, 217, 219, 220–21,
223
crowning in, 191
due date and, 217–18
endorphins in, 187, 216
epidural anesthesia in, 221,
223–25
episiotomy in, 226–27
external fetal monitoring in,
219
fears about, 180–82, 196–97
first stage of, 186–87
inducing or augmenting,
220–24
intravenous access in, 220
massage and, 55
medical intervention in, 177,
184, 218–29
oxytocin in, 189, 205, 209,
216–17, 220, 223
pain medications in, 221,
224–25
placenta in, 193
positions for, 212–15
preparation for, 196–97
questions about, 185
recording your experience,
194–96
second stage of, 187–92
supportive environment for,
207–10
third stage of, 192–93
touch and, 203–6
laughter, 268
leg cramps, 141–42
Levine, Steven, 10

licorice root, 245–46
Lieberman, Michael, 101
lights, dim, 209
listening, conscious, 171–72
lochia, 243

Mann, Stella Terrill, 12
massage, 54–55, 178
  aromas and, 65
  for baby, 262–67
  for back pain during labor,
    206–7
  of perineum, 59–60, 191–92
  postpartum, 240, 241
  self-, 55–60
  unborn baby and, 30, 31, 55
medications, 129–30, 132–33
  for pain, 216, 221, 224–25
meditation, 103–10, 178
  aromas and, 65
  fatherhood and, 279
  mantra, 106–7, 108
  understanding your
    experiences in, 107–10
minerals, 89, 254
miscarriage, 131, 132
misoprostol, 224
moksha, 164, 285, 286–87
mood swings, 144–45, 247
morning sickness, 130–32
  relieving, 78–79, 132–36
Mozart effect, 50
music, 28, 29, 50–51, 262
  aromas and, 65
  during labor, 209
  suggestions for, 53

nasal congestion, 140–41
nausea and vomiting, 130–32
  relieving, 78–79, 132–36

needs
  in Ayurveda, 164, 285–87
  emotions and, 159–61, 164,
    165–68, 169, 282
New Testament, 26–27
nipple stimulation, 217, 223
Nonviolent Communication
  (Rosenberg), 163
nutrition, *see* diet

Ojas, 23
omega-3 and omega-6 fatty acids,
  75, 77, 86–87
ovum (egg), 19–22, 36
oxytocin, 189, 205, 209, 216–17,
  220, 223, 243

pain medications, 216
  in labor, 221, 224–25
Palinsky, Constance, 204
partner, *see* father
pelvic floor toners (Kegel
  exercises), 122–24,
  246–47
pelvic tilts, 117–18
perineum, 117
  crowning and, 191
  episiotomy and, 226–27
  Kegel exercises and, 124,
    246–47
  massage of, 59–60, 191–92
  soothing of, after birth,
    241–43
pigeon pose, 118–19
Pitocin, 219, 220–21, 224
Pitta imbalance, 51, 53, 56
placenta, 22, 25, 36, 40, 132,
  193, 243
Prana, 23
Prechtl, Heinz, 257

pregnancy
    baby's development during,
        19–41
    conception in, 7, 17, 19–26
    diet during, 82–88, 91–93
    health care advisor and, 130,
        147–48
    physical changes in, 129–50
    vitamin and mineral intake
        during, 89
    womb ecology in, 45–69
    yoga in, *see* yoga
progesterone, 25, 137, 138
prostaglandin gel, 223–24
protein, 76, 77, 80, 84–86
psyllium seeds, 245
pungent foods, 76, 78–79

raspberry, 244
Reinold, Emil, 98–99
Robbins, Tom, 158
Rosenberg, Marshall, 161, 163
rotated stomach pose, 121–22

salty foods, 76, 77–78
Samuels, Michael and Nancy,
    13
Saraha, 103
seeing and images, 45, 46, 60–62,
    68, 104
    newborn and, 241, 257, 267
    postpartum, 241
    unborn baby and, 31–32,
        60–62
sensory perception, 5, 48–49, 68
    emotions and, 46–47
    meditation and, 104, 106
    newborn and, 257, 261–68
    postpartum, 241
    see also hearing and sounds;

seeing and images; smelling
    and aromas; tasting and
    flavors; touch and feeling
sexual appetite, 289–90
Shakespeare, William, 273
Shatavari, 253
showers and baths, 209
sight, *see* seeing and images
simple twist exercise, 120–21
sitz bath, 246
sleeping difficulties, 130, 139–40,
    247
    fatherhood and, 279–81
sleeping with your baby,
    259–60
smelling and aromas, 45, 46, 49,
    64–67, 68, 104, 178, 267–68
    diet and, 74
    essential oils, 65–67
    labor and, 208
    newborn and, 241, 257
    postpartum, 241
    in the womb, 32–34, 64–67
sounds, *see* hearing and sounds
sour foods, 76, 77
sperm, 19–20, 21–22
spicy (pungent) foods, 76, 78–79
Spock, Benjamin, 275–76
squat pose, 115–17
stress, 6, 48, 97–101, 197,
    288–89
    fatherhood and, 279
    hormones and, 28, 47, 48, 98,
        103
    images and, 31
    management of, 101–103
    meditation and, 103
    sounds and, 28–29
    touch and, 54
    unborn baby and, 98–101,
        102
    yoga and, 110–11

sudden infant death syndrome (SIDS), 260
sweet foods, 76–77
swelling, 145–46

Tagore, Rabindanath, 95, 300
Taittiriya Upanishad, 71
tasting and flavors, 45, 49, 62–63, 68, 104
  diet and, 74
  newborn and, 257
  six primary tastes, 32, 75, 76–80, 253
  in the womb, 32, 33, 62–63
touch and feeling, 45, 46, 49, 54–60, 68
  during labor, 203–6
  newborn and, 262–67
  in the womb, 29–31, 54–60
  see also massage

Upanishads, 71, 298
urinary tract infections, 146

valerian, 244
Vata imbalance, 51, 53, 56
Vedanta, 299
vegetarian diet, 85
vestibular (balance) system, 29–30
vision, *see* seeing and images
visualization, 10, 14, 15

vitamin supplements, 87–88, 89, 254
  vitamin B$_6$, 134–35

warm pack, 207–8
water, immersion in, 209
water and juice intake, 208, 220
weight gain, 83–84, 132, 289
What Color Is Your Diet? (Heber), 80
Williamson, Marianne, 175
witch hazel, 242, 246
Wolf, Peter, 257
womb, 6, 8
  ecology of, 45–69
  hearing in, 26–29, 50–54
  seeing in, 31–32, 60–62
  smelling in, 32–34, 64–67
  tasting in, 32, 33, 62–63
  touch in, 29–31, 54–60

yoga, 110–25, 178
  aromas and, 65
  butterfly pose, 111–13
  cat and cow pose, 113–15
  child's pose, 119–10
  pelvic tilts, 117–18
  pigeon pose, 118–19
  rotated stomach pose, 121–22
  simple twist, 120–21
  squat pose, 115–17
  unborn baby and, 30, 31, 124–25
Yogananda, Paramhansa, 179

About the Authors

Deepak Chopra's many books have become international bestsellers and classic texts of health and spirituality. Dr. Chopra is founder of the Chopra Center for Well Being in Carlsbad, California.

David Simon, M.D., is the cofounder and medical director of the Chopra Center, and one of the nation's foremost authorities on holistic health care. He is the author of *Vital Energy* and *Return to Wholeness*.

Vicki Abrams, C.C.E., I.B.C.L.C., is the director of the childbirth and yoga programs at the Chopra Center. She is an international board-certified lactation consultant, childbirth educator, doula, and yoga instructor.

The Chopra Center is pleased to offer certification courses to become a Magical Beginnings, Enchanted Lives Birth Educator. For information, please contact us at magical@chopra.com or call (800) 475-4895.

There is nothing inevitable about aging.

THAT IS THE INSPIRING MESSAGE FROM

Deepak Chopra

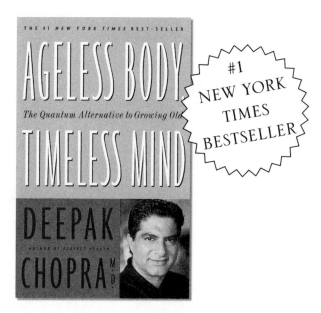

Ageless Body, Timeless Mind
0-517-88212-4 • $14.95 paper • (Canada: $22.95)

"Deepak Chopra is one of the most important healers of our time. Ageless Body, Timeless Mind is a treasure. Having read this book, I feel younger than when I started it."
—MARIANNE WILLIAMSON, author of A Return to Love

"For all those interested in living a long, full life, this book is a valuable resource."
—BERNIE SIEGEL, M.D., author of Life, Love, and Medicine

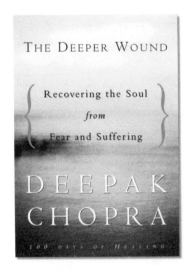

The Deeper Wound
1-4000-4505-3 • $16.00 hardcover
(Canada: $25.00)

Golf for Enlightenment
0-609-60390-6 • $21.00 hardcover
(Canada: $32.00)

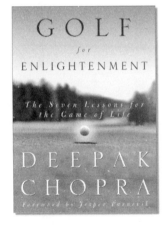

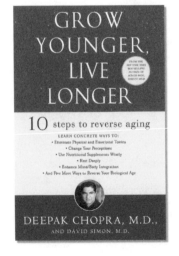

Grow Younger, Live Longer
0-609-81008-1 • $14.00 paper
(Canada: $21.00)

How to Know God
0-609-80523-1 • $14.00 paper
(Canada: $21.00)

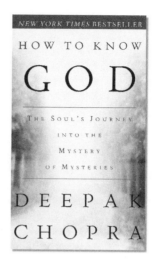

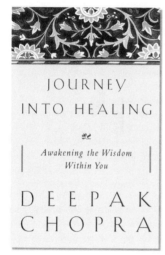

Journey into Healing
1-4000-8069-X • $15.00 paper
(Canada: $22.00)

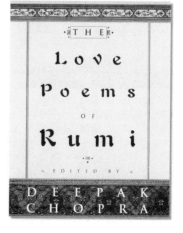

The Love Poems of Rumi
0-609-60243-8 • $12.00 hardcover
(Canada: $18.00)

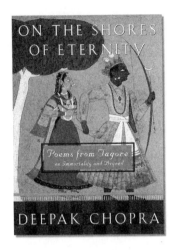

On the Shores of Eternity
0-609-60564-X • $14.00 hardcover
(Canada: $21.00)

The Path to Love
0-609-80135-X • $14.00 paper
(Canada: $18.95)

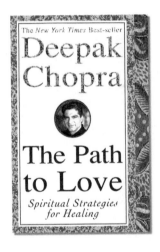

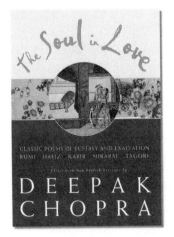

The Soul in Love
0-609-60648-4 • $14.00 hardcover
(Canada: $21.00)

The Spontaneous Fulfillment of Desire
0-609-60042-7 • $25.00 hardcover
(Canada: $35.00)

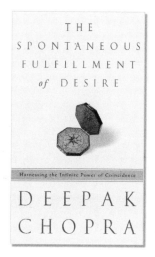

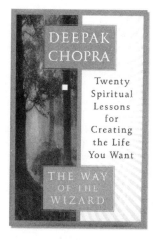

The Way of the Wizard
0-517-70434-X • $16.95 hardcover
(Canada: $25.95)

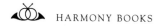 HARMONY BOOKS

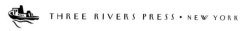 THREE RIVERS PRESS • NEW YORK

Wherever books are sold • www.crownpublishing.com